The
Digest
Diet
Dining Out Guide

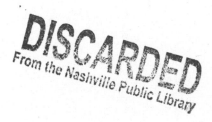

The
Digest
Diet
Dining Out Guide

Follow the breakthrough diet on the go!

- Fat Releasing Fast Food
- Best Restaurant Meals for Each Phase
- Portable Shakes and Snacks

LIZ VACCARIELLO

Editor-in-Chief of *Reader's Digest* and author of
the *New York Times* bestseller ***The Digest Diet***

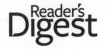

The Reader's Digest Association, Inc.
New York, NY/Montreal

A READER'S DIGEST BOOK

Copyright © 2013 The Reader's Digest Association, Inc.

Library of Congress Cataloging-in-Publication Data
Vaccariello, Liz.
  The digest diet eating-out guide : follow the breakthrough diet on the go! / by Liz Vaccariello, editor-in-chief of Reader's Digest.
      p. cm.
  ISBN 978-1-62145-011-5 (trade pbk. : alk. paper) -- ISBN 978-1-62145-000-9 (direct mail pbk. : alk. paper) -- ISBN 978-1-62145-012-2 (e pub : alk. paper)
  1. Reducing diets. 2. Low-fat diet. 3. Nutrition. 4. Self-care, Health. I. Title.
  RM222.2V2543 2013
  613.2'5--dc23

                          2012032502

ISBN 978-1-62145-011-5

We are committed to both the quality of our products and the service we provide to our customers. We value your comments, so please feel free to contact us.

          The Reader's Digest Association, Inc.
          Adult Trade Publishing
          44 South Broadway
          White Plains, NY 10601

For more Reader's Digest products and information, visit our website:
          www.rd.com (in the United States)

Printed in the United States of America

1 3 5 7 9 10 8 6 4 2

NOTE TO OUR READERS
The information in this book should not be substituted for, or used to alter, medical therapy without your doctor's advice. For a specific health problem, consult your physician for guidance.
Mention of specific companies, organizations, or products in this book does not imply endorsement by the author or publisher, nor does mention of specific companies, organizations, or products imply that they endorse this book, its author or the publisher.
Internet addresses and telephone numbers given in this book were accurate at the time it went to press.

The Digest Diet

Go online for **EXCLUSIVE** success tools and tricks… **and it's all FREE!**

- **Guaranteed motivation** with community and support

- **Inspiring videos** full of savvy tips and insider advice from other Digest Diet participants

- **The latest news and studies** on fat releasing foods, moves, and attitudes, plus updates from the experts

- **Even more delicious recipes** starring your favorite fat releasers to keep you feeling full and fabulous

- **Food and fitness journals** to help you reach your goal

- **The best jokes** and funny stuff to get you to "laugh it off" when you need it

readersdigest.com/digestdiet

facebook.com/digestdiet

Contents

My **greatest joy** as an editor is knowing that the information and advice I bring to readers makes a real difference in their lives. That is why I am thrilled about the success of the Digest Diet. Every day, I hear from readers like you who have lost weight and improved their health by following this eating and lifestyle plan.

To develop the Digest Diet, the *Reader's Digest* staff and I did what we do best. We sorted through all the information we could find on weight loss success and condensed it into simple, easy-to-follow advice. No weight loss gimmicks and fads, just the delicious foods and everyday habits that lead to results. Then we recruited 12 men and women who put the Digest Diet to the test. In just 21 days, they lost a collective 151 pounds. Our biggest loser, Joe Rinaldi, had struggled to lose weight for years; on the Digest Diet, he dropped 26 pounds and found that he had less knee pain and more energy and confidence. Not only that, testers reported feeling less sluggish, sleeping better, and enjoying life more.

For those 21 days, we asked our testers to cook all of their meals. But as a busy working mom, I know that's not realistic for everyone. And as much as I enjoy cooking and eating at home with my husband and daughters, I don't believe you should have to give up dinners out in order to stay on a diet.

Thankfully, nutrition information is more readily available at restaurants these days, but it can still be pretty confusing to figure out which items on the menu are healthiest. So for this guide, the *Reader's Digest* staff and I combed through menus from dozens of restaurants, and picked out fat releasing foods. We then combined them into meals that you can choose whenever you're eating away from home.

If you are new to the Digest Diet, be sure to read Part 1 of this book for an overview of the plan. You may also want to pick up a copy of the original book, *The Digest Diet*, which is filled with information, recipes, and a 21-day meal plan. While you're on Phase 1, the 4-day Fast Release, I suggest that you avoid eating out. Restaurant offerings for Phase 1 are extremely limited, although we have picked out a few that come closest to our guidelines. This book is best for readers in Phases 2 and 3.

Please promise me that you won't be hard on yourself if a meal isn't perfect. I am all about striving to be the best that you can be while accepting that the road to success can be bumpy. You may pick a restaurant, only to find that the menu has very little that fits into the Digest Diet. Or the meal that you carefully ordered is not the same as what comes on your plate. The most important thing is to stick to the diet as closely as you can and get right back into your diet the next meal. That's what I do each and every day, and that's how I keep my weight in check.

Now get out there and start eating!

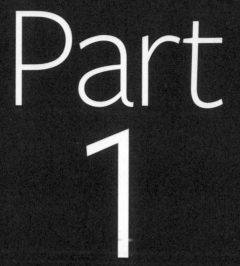

Part 1

The Digest
Version of
the Digest Diet

At its heart, the Digest Diet is about foods that you can enjoy without guilt—foods that actually stimulate your body to release fat. I was excited to discover fat releasers in many of my favorite foods, even chocolate. Later in this section and throughout this book, we'll show you where to find these fat releasing foods when you're eating out.

But you also need to be aware of the sneaky fat increasers in our environment that cause your body to want to hang on to fat. We sorted them into categories I call the "three E's"—eating, environment, and exercise. You can read about these in more detail in *The Digest Diet* and *The Digest Diet Cookbook*, but when you're dining out, you need to be particularly aware of these fat increasers:

PORTIONS. After 20 years as a health journalist, I thought I was savvy about supersized restaurant portions. But as I researched meals for this book, even I was shocked to find out how big restaurant entrées are and how many calories they contain. I'm talking meals that are at least 800 to some well over 1,000. Once you add in an appetizer, drink, and dessert, a meal can easily add up to more calories than you need for the entire day.

ENVIRONMENT. Did you know that restaurants use subtle tricks with lighting, music, plate size, and where items appear on the menu to get you to eat more food? While there's not much you

FAT INCREASERS—THE 3 E'S

Eating	Environment	Exercise
Too much food	Too much sitting	Too little variety
Too little food	Too much thinking	Too little effort
Too little satisfaction	Too much or too little sleep	Too little enjoyment
	Too much pollution	
	Too little joy	

can do about these, just being aware of them can keep you—not your subconscious—in charge of what and how much you eat.

FAKE FOOD. Too much restaurant food is highly processed and filled with fat, sugar, and salt. That makes it extremely appealing and very hard to stop eating.

LACK OF NUTRIENTS. Restaurant meals can be lacking in key micronutrients that help regulate body fat and appetite, such as calcium, vitamin C, zinc, magnesium, and vitamin E. So this book guides you to the proper portions of foods that are rich in nutrients.

● THE THREE PHASES OF THE DIGEST DIET

When we created the Digest Diet, we divided it into three phases for maximum fat burning. The first phase, the 4-day Fast Release, is designed to shed fat quickly, with two nutrient-rich shakes and a generous bowl of soup each day. I discourage eating out during Phase 1, since it's virtually impossible to find restaurant shakes and soups that have the right balance of fat releasing ingredients. For those times when you have to be on the go during Phase 1, though, I've called out a few shakes and soups that come closest to meeting our Digest Diet standards.

The Digest Diet Shake: Take It to Go!

● **Phase 1 (Fast Release):** In a blender, combine ¾ cup (6 ounces) nonfat yogurt, ¼ cup light coconut milk, 3 tablespoons nonfat milk powder, 2 teaspoons honey, ½ teaspoon vanilla extract, 4 ice cubes, fruit/fiber (choose 1 from the list below), healthy fat (choose 1 from the list below), and flavoring, if desired (choose from the list below). Note that the shake is minimally sweet on purpose to keep you from getting hungry too soon, so please don't add more honey.

● **Phase 2 (Fade Away):** Reduce the light coconut milk to 2 tablespoons and add 2 tablespoons water. Also, reduce your healthy fat option to 1 teaspoon (or ¼ avocado).

FRUIT/FIBER (choose 1)
1 banana
1 apple (peeled and cored) + 1 tablespoon flaxseed meal
8 strawberries (fresh or frozen) + 1 tablespoon flaxseed meal

4 ounces mixed frozen berries (¾ to 1 cup, depending on the berries' size) + 1 tablespoon flaxseed meal
¾ cup seedless red grapes (10 large) + 1 tablespoon flaxseed meal. Omit the honey.
1 tangerine or small orange + 1 tablespoon flaxseed meal

HEALTHY FATS (choose 1)
½ avocado
1 tablespoon natural peanut butter
1 tablespoon raw or regular almond butter
1 tablespoon tahini
1 tablespoon sunflower seed butter

FLAVORINGS (choose none, 1, or both)
1 teaspoon unsweetened cocoa powder
¼ teaspoon ground cinnamon

FAT RELEASERS: Yogurt, coconut milk, fruit/fiber, healthy fats, honey

THE DIGEST DIET... AT A GLANCE

Phase 1 (Fast Release): Days 1 through 4

- Drink two shakes a day as meals .
- Eat one crunchy snack a day (see page 7 for snack suggestions).
- Have soup for one of your meals .

Phase 2 (Fade Away): Days 5 through 14

- Have one shake a day.
- Go lean (proteins) and green (veggies) at meals.
- Choose MUFAs and omega-3 PUFAs for your healthy fats.
- Snack twice a day.
- Enjoy a glass of red wine or a bunch of red grapes at dinner.

Phase 3 (Finish Strong): Days 15 through 21

- Choose meals carefully to have the right balance of different types of foods.
- Continue to snack twice a day.
- Continue to enjoy a glass of red wine with dinner.
- Enjoy a dessert or favorite treat once a week .

Fundamentals for all phases

- Include fat releasers at every meal and snack.
- Thrive with five—fiber, protein, vitamin C, calcium, and dairy—by including them at most meals.
- Before each meal or snack, drink a big glass of water with a few generous squeezes of fresh lemon, lime, or orange.
- Eat three servings of fat-free, low-fat, or reduced-fat dairy each day.

Phase 2 Fade Away includes one shake a day that has slightly less fat than the Fast Release Shake. I recommend that you make and bring your own when you're eating away from home (see the recipe on page 3) since you're unlikely to find an exact fat-releasing match on a restaurant menu. Lunch and dinner consist of lean protein plus vegetables, especially leafy greens. This combination is recommended in Phase 2 to maximize fat release and boost metabolism while supplying your body with important nutrients. You also can add a 4-ounce glass of wine at dinner.

Phase 3 Finish Strong is meant to be your maintenance phase; in order to keep the weight off, you'll want to keep eating this way for the rest of your life. In this phase, you can add some carbohydrates, ideally in the form of whole grains like brown rice or whole-grain bread. Sadly, this is an area where most restaurants are lacking. Where whole-grain choices were available, we've pointed them out; where they were not, we came as close as possible. Another option is to bring your own whole grain to supplement your restaurant meal—see our Whole Grains To Go Kit on page 10 for some easy, portable ideas. Or you can just skip the carbs altogether; it's certainly fine to have some Phase 2 meals during Phase 3. If you do add carbs, you'll generally need to reduce the amount of meat or other protein you're eating in order to make sure you don't overdo your calories.

In Phase 3 you can enjoy a dessert or favorite treat once a week. Once you start seeing the results of eating the Digest Diet way, though, I think you'll find that you simply don't want restaurant desserts anymore. Instead, here's what I suggest: Have fruit if it's available. Then grab a fork and have a small taste of a dessert ordered by someone at your table.

Each phase includes at least one daily snack (about 100 to 150 calories) of foods that supply protein, fiber, and vitamin C. Because you're not likely to find the right combination of fat releasing nutrients in snack portions on a restaurant menu, I recommend that you create your own. See the chart on the opposite for some ideas.

● DINING OUT ON THE DIGEST DIET

As the *Reader's Digest* staff and I pored over nearly 100 restaurant menus, we were struck by the differences in Digest Diet–friendly offerings. Some chains have so many veggie and protein choices that we could have put together dozens of meals. Others, especially those that sell fast food or pizza, are extremely limited. That's why my most important piece of advice to you is this: Put together the best meal you can under the circumstances, using our Digest Diet guidelines. In general, I still encourage you to prepare meals at home as much as possible to have control over what you eat. Also, if you know your meal at a restaurant is light in fiber, vitamin C, or other fat releasers, you can make up for it in your next meals at home.

We followed these general parameters for Digest Diet meals:

- 425–450 calories
- Protein, dairy, calcium, vitamin C, and fiber in most meals
- 4 ounces lean meat or poultry, or 6 ounces fish or seafood
- At least 2 cups of vegetables

Even though I give you a calorie range for each meal, I don't want you to go crazy counting calories. The meals in this book were chosen to come close to the recommended range so that you

PORTABLE SNACKS

Mix and match! Choose one food from each category below to create a Digest Diet snack you can take anywhere.

For fiber:

1 cup broccoli florets

4 mini bell peppers

4 cucumber wedges

1 cup green beans

1 single-serve packet of baby carrots or celery sticks

1 small vegetable snack tray (no dip)

1 high-fiber cracker (see the list on page 10)

1 small apple (Phase 3 only)

1 small pear (Phase 3 only)

For protein:

1 mini-cheese*

5.3- to 6-ounce container plain fat-free yogurt

1 tablespoon nuts or seeds

2 tablespoons hummus

½ cup in-pod edamame

For vitamin C:

10 grape or cherry tomatoes

1 cup cauliflower florets

½ cup sugar snap peas

1 cup mixed vegetable juice

2 clementines (Phase 3 only)

1 kiwifruit (Phase 3 only)

1 orange (Phase 3 only)

½ cup cantaloupe (Phase 3 only)

½ grapefruit (Phase 3 only)

½ cup mango chunks (Phase 3 only)

½ cup papaya chunks (Phase 3 only)

½ cup berries (Phase 3 only)

*Choose single-serving reduced-fat cheeses like The Laughing Cow Mini Babybel Light, The Laughing Cow Light, Les Petites Fermieres Reduced-Fat Cheddar Cheese Sticks, Sargento Reduced-Fat Colby-Jack Stick, Polly-O 2% Mozzarella & Cheddar Cheese Twist.

don't need to do the math. I do encourage you, however, to master portion sizes. Because portions vary from restaurant to restaurant and even from chef to chef at the same restaurant, you'll want to be able to eyeball your plate to make sure you're following our portion recommendations. The box on the opposite page can help you match portions to common restaurant items.

Sometimes my family is embarrassed to go out to eat with me. Why? I often ask endless questions about how dishes are made (poor waitstaff!). Here's a little advice: Find out as much as you can before you place your order. Then, use the following shortcuts to Digest Diet eating that I've developed after visiting hundreds of restaurants and eating thousands of meals away from home:

1. Spy on neighboring tables to see how much food is on their plates. I've made lots of new friends that way, once I explain why I'm staring at their plate! I also ask the waitstaff if the restaurant portions tend to be large, medium, or small, although my idea of small and large often is different from theirs. When you're asking about how a dish is served, remember that those served "family style" are meant to feed at least two people and usually more.

2. Choose your veggies before selecting your protein. Raw or steamed are best so that you can avoid unwanted fat increasers. Otherwise, lightly sautéed or stir-fried veggies are a suitable alternative; just watch the portion size because they're higher in calories. I have to warn you, though—in several chains, lettuce and tomato will be your only options.

3. Mix and match to reach 2 cups of vegetables. You can do this a few different ways: Order a large portion of one vegetable, pair a salad with a veggie side dish, or enjoy a large salad. Sometimes

PORTION GUIDE FOR DINING OUT

1 tablespoon	Single-serve mustard or mayo packet, small paper ketchup cup
2 tablespoons	Level salad bar serving spoon, salad dressing ladle
¼ cup	Plastic salad dressing cup, metal sauce cup, rounded salad bar serving spoon
½ cup	Round ice cream scoop
1 cup	Diner/coffee shop mug; small to-go coffee cup
4 ounces (meat, poultry)	Slice of bread (the type in a grocery store loaf)
6 ounces (fish)	Slice of thicker country-style bread

I mine the menu looking for vegetables that are listed as part of an entrée and then I ask for a small plate of just those veggies. When I'm faced with a menu that doesn't list vegetable side dishes, like some of the sandwich shops and pizza places in this book, I ask for a plate piled high with every possible vegetable they have. Sadly, sometimes it's just a big pile of lettuce, as you'll see in several of our sample meals.

4. Ask how dishes are prepared and listen carefully for fat increasers such as butter and cream. Find out whether a dish can be modified to be served without the high-calorie extras.

5. Always ask for dressing and sauces on the side, or, better yet, do without them. Almost all will have fat, sugar, or other fat increasers.

6. Manage carbs. When you're in Phase 2, your plate should have just vegetables and protein, no rice, pasta, bread, or potatoes. Ask the waitstaff to leave these off your plate. Your Phase 3 carb portion is ½ cup of a cooked grain or one slice of bread. Whole grain always is best, but our sample meals may include a small

WHOLE GRAINS TO GO KIT

No whole grains on the menu? These high-fiber wraps and crackers keep well in your purse or car.

Wraps and flatbreads

Aladdin Low-Carb Wheat Wrap

Damascus Bakeries Roll-Up (flax, wheat)

Flatout Flatbread (multigrain with flax, whole grain white)

Flatout Flatbread Light (original)

La Tortilla Factory Smart & Delicious Large Size Tortilla (whole wheat)

La Tortilla Factory Smart & Delicious Soft Wraps (multigrain)

La Tortilla Factory Smart & Delicious Extra Virgin Olive Oil Soft Wraps

South Beach Diet (whole wheat)

Tumaro's Gourmet Tortillas (multigrain)

Crackers (one serving is two crackers)

Wasa crackers

Finn Crisp Plus

RyKrisp Multigrain

Kavli Five Grain

portion of white rice, potato, or other carbs when whole grains aren't available. I also keep a Whole Grains To Go Kit (see the opposite page) in my purse or car, just in case there's nothing for me to choose on the menu.

7. Think lean with proteins. Choose lower-fat cuts such as sirloin. Remove the skin from chicken before eating. Order fish grilled. Portions will be too big most of the time (see page 9 for a portion guide), so trim them down to the right size and bring the rest home. Enjoy beans instead of or in addition to beef or poultry.

8. Look for fruit on the side dish and dessert menus, especially if vegetables are lacking. In Phase 2, the ideal is to stick to vegetables rather than fruit because some fruits are relatively high in sugar, but of course fruits have other health benefits and deliver many of the same nutrients and fat releasers as vegetables do.

9. For calcium and dairy, order a cup of fat-free milk or a cappuccino or latte made with fat-free milk whenever they're on the menu. Otherwise, include up to an ounce of cheese.

10. Be smart about foods and portions—it's up to you to manage your meal. Although we tell you how much to eat based on information on restaurant menus and websites, what you get on your plate might be completely different.

● FAT RELEASING CUISINES

Fat releasing is universal! Every traditional cuisine features fat releasing ingredients—though sadly their restaurant versions sometimes swap them out for fat increasers. Here are a few tips on what to look for at different types of restaurants.

American/Steakhouse

American cuisine is no longer just meat and potatoes, even at classic steakhouses. With influences from around the world, American restaurants have taken the best of international fare and added a uniquely American interpretation. Sadly, this isn't always best for our collective health, as American restaurant fare tends to be high in fat and served in overly large portions. The appetizer menu—filled with fried fare and creamy dips—is a particular fat increaser for followers of the Digest Diet. On the fat releasing side, you have a lot to choose from, especially salads, grilled meat and chicken, vegetable side dishes, and fresh fruit.

In Phase 2, your best bets are:

- Grilled chicken or steak Caesar salad (no dressing or croutons)
- Grilled or roasted steak, chicken, or turkey (4 ounces) with two vegetable side dishes
- Shrimp or tuna (6 ounces) with two vegetable side dishes

In Phase 3, reduce your protein portion by 1 to 2 ounces, and add ½ cup of rice or potato or a whole-wheat roll. Leave room in your meal for a 4-ounce glass of red wine or sangria if you're dining at a restaurant that has a bar. You're also likely to have access to milk or a coffee drink with milk, such as cappuccino, but there are no guarantees that the milk will be fat-free.

Chinese

A lot of people tell me that they're hungry an hour or so after eating a Chinese meal. So as I gathered information on Chinese restaurants, I didn't expect to find a lot of fat increasers. You can imagine how shocked I was to learn just how many calories are in some of my favorite dishes. I looked more closely and discovered a few things. First, cooking food quickly in a wok requires a lot of oil. Second, the sauces chefs add to dishes often have a lot of sugar. And, most important, even though the portion served looks like it should be for one person, it has enough calories for two.

Here's the good news—Chinese food is really easy to customize since a lot of dishes are cooked to order. Be as specific as possible about wanting your food cooked with only a little oil or in broth instead. In Phase 2, your best bets are:

- Stir-fried chicken or tofu with vegetables (2 cups) (no rice) with hot and sour or egg drop soup (1 cup)
- Steamed beef, pork, or shrimp with vegetables (2½ cups)
- Chinese chicken salad (2 cups)

If you find the steamed dishes too plain, spice them up with Digest Diet–friendly hot chili pepper, a dash of soy sauce, and a couple drops of sesame oil. In Phase 3, eat a little less meat and add ½ cup of plain rice, preferably brown.

Deli/Sandwich Shop

Here's why I like delis and sandwich shops for dishing up Digest Diet meals—much of the food they serve is totally à la carte, so I can put together whatever combination of protein and vegetables

I'm in the mood for. Most vegetarian soups—including vegetable, lentil, or black bean—are usually fine for Phase 1. They usually have at least one whole-grain option for Phase 3. And they have lots of innovative combos and salads.

But that's where they often diverge from the Digest Diet. Look closely at deli salads and you're likely to notice a shine to them or a white coating. It's extra fat, usually oil or mayonnaise, a classic fat increaser. So I encourage you to stick with plainer stuff rather than prepared salads.

In Phase 2, your best bets are:

- Roast beef, ham, turkey or chicken breast (4 ounces) with vegetables or fruit (2 cups)
- Chef's salad (no dressing)
- Beef chili with a side salad

In Phase 3, reduce your protein portion by 1 to 2 ounces, and add a whole-grain bread or roll.

Diner/Coffee Shop

I love diners and coffee shops because they have a little bit of everything on the menu, including breakfast dishes, salads, soups, sandwiches, entrées, and multicourse meals. But portion sizes vary from modest to huge, depending on the restaurant, so you have to get a sense of how much typically is served before you place your order. There's nothing I love more than a bargain, but the calories in a complete meal are not worth the price. Order à la carte or hit the salad bar instead.

In Phase 2, your best bets are:

- Scrambled eggs or omelette (2 eggs) with vegetables and fruit on the side
- Salad of mixed raw vegetables (2 cups) topped with grilled chicken or sliced sandwich meat (4 ounces)
- Meatloaf or burger patty (4 ounces) with cooked vegetables and/or salad on the side

In Phase 3, reduce your protein portion by 1 to 2 ounces and add ½ cup rice, ½ plain baked potato, or a whole-wheat roll.

Fast Food/Burgers

Fast-food outlets have improved a great deal in recent years. Many chains offer one or more salads, low-fat or even fat-free milk, apple slices, and some smaller-sized dishes. I ended up spending hours playing with online calorie and nutrition counters that let me customize my meal by taking off and adding different ingredients and then tracking the change in calories.

That said, variety in vegetables is lacking, you may not find a large enough portion of vegetables to balance your meal, and it's virtually impossible to find a whole grain to sub in for Phase 3. Also, you may have to create your own "mix and match" meal from several menu items (we'll tell you how).

In Phase 2, your best bet is a hamburger patty or grilled chicken breast (no bread or sauce) with a garden salad on the side. In Phase 3, add half a bun.

Italian and Pizza

The carb-centric nature of Italian-American fare can make Digest Diet dining a bit challenging, especially at pizza joints where your only Phase 2 choice may be an assortment of vegetable and grated cheeses typically used as pizza toppings—not very satisfying! So I recommend skipping them in Phase 2. In Phase 3, you can enjoy an occasional slice of veggie pizza.

You'll find more to choose from at casual dining restaurants. Italian restaurants tend to serve a lot of food, often family-style, so you'll need to use your portion management skills to avoid overdoing it. Ask if foods can be grilled, steamed or very lightly sautéed rather than breaded and fried. Italians are known for their wine, so enjoy a 4-ounce glass when you can!

In Phase 2, your best bets are:

- Veggie antipasto platter (no dressing) with 8 cubes (2 ounces) of cheese
- Roasted garlic chicken (4 ounces) with minestrone soup and vegetables on the side
- Mussels in tomato sauce (2 cups) with vegetables on the side

Japanese

I always feel so good after eating Japanese food. Most foods on the menu are really healthy, so it's easy to put together Digest Diet meals. With the exception of a few fried classics—katsu and tempura come to mind—and mayonnaise-y sushi rolls, Japanese foods are prepared without much fat, so they tend to be low in calories. Just ask your teppanyaki grill chef to go easy on the oil when he sautés your meat and veggies.

The Japanese appetizer menu has veggie dishes that I almost never see anywhere else, such as seaweed salads, spinach with sesame seeds, and marinated radishes. Be sure to ask if the restaurant has brown rice. It has become so popular that some chefs offer it as an option in their sushi rolls. Most Japanese restaurants are not part of nationwide chains, so the offerings will vary from restaurant to restaurant.

In Phase 2, your best bets are:

- Teppanyaki steak and vegetables (2½ cups)
- Teriyaki chicken or salmon (4–6 ounces) with seaweed salad and steamed broccoli on the side
- Sashimi (8 pieces) with edamame and pickled radishes

Mexican

Authentic Mexican cuisine is filled with fat releasers from the obvious (healthy fats in the avocado, fiber in the beans, calcium in the cheese) to the not-so-obvious (moles made with cocoa, salsas and sauces made with vitamin C–rich vegetables and fruits, sangrias made with red wine). But the Tex-Mex versions we often find in restaurants in the United States tend to heap on refined carbs like rice and tortillas and grill with a generous amount of oil, and the portions are huge!

In Phase 2, your best approach is à la carte. You can create your own combination meals from grilled items such as fajita vegetables, chicken, and beef; salad veggies; beans; and salsas. Dishes on the menu often have unexpected extras such as rice, sour cream, and fried tortilla chips, so tell the kitchen to leave them off your meal. Your best bets are:

- Chicken or steak fajitas (4 ounces meat) with grilled vegetables, guacamole (¼ cup) and salsa but no tortilla
- Chicken mole with salad and guacamole (¼ cup)

   • Bean burrito with lettuce, tomatoes, pico de gallo, and grated cheese (2 tablespoons) but no rice or tortilla

You have a bit more flexibility in Phase 3 to add a tortilla or some rice, but try not to go overboard with your portions! And look for more unusual vegetables to try like jicama (a crunchy root vegetable that is full of fiber) and nopales (the leaf of the prickly pear cactus, which is rich in vitamin C).

● HOW TO USE THIS BOOK

In Part 2, you'll find a list of national restaurant chains. For each restaurant, I've given you sample meals to order as specified or use as a template for ordering other items from the menu. The meals fit the Phase 2 guidelines, with suggested modifications to adapt them to Phase 3.

While I used the most up-to-date information from restaurant menus and websites, offerings change frequently and websites are not always kept updated. So don't be surprised if you find suitable menu items that I didn't mention or foods that are no longer on the menu. You may want to plan ahead by using information on the restaurant website—we provide a URL for each chain and call out those restaurants with particularly robust nutrition tools.

I also highlighted the fat releasing foods in each meal. I discovered that some restaurant menus have more fat releasers than others. If you'd like to find your own, here's a list of the fat releasing foods and nutrients I identified in my research:

● VITAMIN C

Vegetables
- Asparagus
- Bell peppers
- Broccoli
- Broccoli rabe
- Brussels sprouts
- Cabbage
- Cauliflower
- Escarole
- Garlic
- Greens (collards, mustard, turnip)
- Kale
- Kohlrabi
- Onions
- Peas, sugar snap
- Spinach
- Squash, summer and winter
- Sweet potatoes

Fruits
- Cantaloupe
- Grapefruit and fresh juice
- Kiwifruit
- Lemons
- Limes
- Mango
- Oranges and fresh juice
- Papaya
- Pineapple
- Raspberries
- Strawberries
- Tomatoes

● CALCIUM AND DAIRY

Dairy
- Buttermilk
- Cheese (cheddar, cottage, cream, feta, gruyère, mozzarella, Parmesan, provolone, ricotta, Swiss)
- Milk
- Yogurt

Nuts and seeds
- Almonds or almond butter
- Brazil nuts
- Roasted sesame seeds or sesame butter

Vegetables
- Bok choy
- Broccoli
- Broccoli rabe
- Greens (collards, dandelion, mustard, and turnip)
- Kale
- Spinach
- Watercress

● PROTEIN

Beans and legumes
- Baby lima beans
- Black beans
- Chickpeas
- Lentils
- Soybeans
- White beans

Dairy (see above)

Grains
- Barley
- Couscous, whole-wheat
- Oats

Nuts and seeds
- Almonds and almond butter
- Hazelnuts
- Peanuts and peanut butter
- Pistachios
- Pumpkin, sunflower, squash, or watermelon seeds

Poultry and eggs
- Chicken
- Eggs
- Turkey

Meats (lean cuts)
- Beef
- Pork
- Veal

Fish
- Anchovies, fresh
- Cod
- Crab
- Halibut
- Lobster
- Salmon, canned and fresh
- Sardines, canned and fresh
- Shrimp
- Tuna, canned and fresh

● FIBER

Fruits
- Avocado
- Blackberries
- Plums
- Raspberries
- Tomatoes (fresh and sun-dried)

Legumes
- Beans
- Chickpeas
- Lentils
- Peas

Grains
- Barley
- Couscous, whole-wheat
- Rice, brown
- Oats

Nuts and seeds
- Almonds
- Brazil nuts
- Flaxseed and flaxseed meal
- Pecans
- Pistachios
- Sesame seeds
- Sunflower seeds

Vegetables
- Artichoke
- Broccoli rabe
- Greens (mustard and turnip)
- Lettuce
- Radishes
- Vinegar

● POLYUNSATURATED FATS (PUFAS) AND MONOUNSATURATED FATS (MUFAS)*

- Avocado
- Coconut milk
- Nuts, seeds, and nut butters, particularly flax, walnut, and sunflower
- Olive oil
- Salmon
- Sardines
- Soybean oil
- Sunflower oil

● RESVERATROL

- Red grapes
- Red wine
- Spanish peanuts

● VINEGAR

● COCONUT OIL

● QUINOA

● HONEY

● COCOA**

*I didn't make a special effort to include these in your restaurant meal since chefs commonly use them in cooking.

**In restaurants, you'll mostly find cocoa in high-fat, high-calorie desserts that aren't suitable on the Digest Diet. To satisfy my chocolate cravings, I'll take a taste of someone else's chocolate dessert. I also keep a small stash of high-quality dark chocolate and nibble on a small amount when I need a treat.

Part
2

Release Fat
at Your Favorite
Restaurant

You should see my office. My staff and I combed through dozens of menus from national restaurant chains to put together a comprehensive guide to help you release fat at your favorite spot. For each restaurant, we give you a bit of information on the chain, tell you where to find nutrition information, and then offer several sample meals or snacks. Our recommendations are based on menu items available at the time we went to print and our best estimates of what and how much is served. Remember, portions or ingredients may vary in individual locations. So you need to train your eyes—and your stomach—to recognize what an appropriate serving of food is.

In some chains, as you'll see, in order to get the right balance of lean protein and fat releasing veggies, you need to do some mixing and matching of foods from different menu items. Some restaurants are happy to accommodate these sorts of requests; others may charge extra or even require you to pay for two dishes (even if, for instance, you are only eating half the ingredients in each). Needless to say, these restaurants aren't the best choices for Digest Diet dining, but we've included them in case you find yourself stuck. Even if a restaurant proves unhelpful, remember that "not perfect" is okay; one indulgent meal won't derail your results. Just stick as closely to the Digest Diet guidelines as you can.

APPLEBEE'S

- 1,990 restaurants in 49 states
- (888) 592-7753; www.applebees.com

This casual dining giant has an extensive menu with plenty of foods to choose from. Its long-standing relationship with Weight Watchers means that you'll find a number of dishes that are controlled in calories and portion size, but they typically don't have the right balance of nutrients for the Digest Diet. You may want to mix and match foods from different dishes, and ask to have fat increasing ingredients left out, to get just the meal you want. You can download nutrition information on the full menu through a link in the bottom section of the website.

> ### Fun
> ### Fat Fact
> The resveratrol in an occasional glass of red wine helps release fat, as well as fight inflammation and lower the risk of heart disease.

● WARNING! Fat Increaser Ahead

When you eat, the various hormones and compounds that are produced by your GI tract take about 20 minutes to reach your brain. Slow down your meal by ordering one course at a time to give your stomach time to signal that it's full before you overeat.

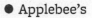

Roasted Garlic Sirloin

FAT RELEASERS: beef, garlic, vegetables
- **Phase 2:** Order the Roasted Garlic Sirloin without creamed spinach or potatoes. Have an order of seasonal vegetables on the side.
- **Phase 3:** Reduce the steak by 1 ounce, or about 2 tablespoons, and add ½ plain baked potato.

Weight Watchers Cabernet Mushroom Sirloin

FAT RELEASERS: beef, red wine, onions, broccoli
- **Phase 2:** Ask for the Cabernet Mushroom Sirloin topped with grilled onions and with the broccoli side dish only.
- **Phase 3:** Reduce the beef by 1 ounce, or about 2 tablespoons. Add ½ plain baked potato.

House Sirloin

FAT RELEASERS: beef, lettuce, vegetables, fruit
- **Phase 2:** Eat ½ order (3.5 ounces) of the House Sirloin with no toppings or side dishes. Instead, ask for the Applebee's House Salad without dressing, and order fresh fruit.
- **Phase 3:** Reduce the sirloin to ⅓ order (about 2.5 ounces). Add 1 slice of wheat bread.

Hamburger Patty

FAT RELEASERS: beef, vegetables, fruit
- **Phase 2:** Ask for a plain burger patty with no bun or sides. Get an order of seasonal vegetables and an order of fresh fruit instead.
- **Phase 3:** Add ½ cup of red beans and rice.

Grilled Steak Caesar Salad

FAT RELEASERS: beef, lettuce
- **Phase 2:** Order the Grilled Chicken Caesar Salad without dressing or croutons, but substitute steak for the chicken.
- **Phase 3:** Reduce the steak by 1 ounce, or about 2 tablespoons, and add a slice of wheat bread.

Grilled Chicken Caesar Salad

FAT RELEASERS: chicken, lettuce, vegetables
- **Phase 2:** Order the Grilled Chicken Caesar Salad with no dressing or croutons. Add a side of seasonal vegetables.
- **Phase 3:** Cut out 1 ounce, or about 2 tablespoons, of chicken. Add 1 small roll.

Oriental Chicken Salad

FAT RELEASERS: chicken, greens, almonds, fruit

● **Phase 2:** Get ½ order of the Oriental Chicken Salad with no dressing or crispy noodles but ask for grilled chicken instead of fried, and a side of fresh fruit.

● **Phase 3:** Reduce the chicken by 1 ounce, or about 2 tablespoons, and add ½ cup of rice.

Weight Watchers Grilled Jalapeño-Lime Shrimp

FAT RELEASERS: shrimp, chile peppers, lime, zucchini, onion, bell pepper, tomato

● **Phase 2:** Order the Weight Watchers Grilled Jalapeño-Lime Shrimp with no rice. Ask for a side of fresh fruit.

● **Phase 3:** Reduce the shrimp by 1 ounce, or about 2 tablespoons, and add ½ cup of rice.

Blackened Tilapia

FAT RELEASERS: fish, lettuce, vegetables

● **Phase 2:** Order the Blackened Tilapia with no sides and one Applebee's House Salad without dressing.

● **Phase 3:** Reduce the tilapia by 1 ounce, or about 2 tablespoons. Add ½ plain baked potato.

Orange Glazed Salmon

FAT RELEASERS: salmon, orange, vegetables

● **Phase 2:** Order the Orange Glazed Salmon with no sides, plus a side of seasonal vegetables.

● **Phase 3:** Reduce the salmon by 1 ounce, or about 2 tablespoons. Add ½ cup of rice.

● **WARNING! Fat Increaser Ahead**

When you're looking at nutrition information on the menu or on a restaurant's website, how can you tell if vegetable dishes are made with added fat, sauce, or sugar if the information is not readily available? Look at calories, and, if available, fat. A serving of plain cooked vegetables should have no more than about 30 calories and zero fat. More calories or fat means that something has been added.

ARBY'S

- More than 3,500 restaurants
- (679) 514-4100; www.arbys.com

Arby's is known for its beef sandwiches and has few veggies and fruit to offer. Create your own meal by picking different items to combine, for example, the beef from a sandwich plus the makings of a salad. A nutrition information chart is accessible through the food section of the website.

> **Fun Fat Fact**
> Our cows have been on a diet, too. They're bred to be skinnier, so today's beef is much leaner than it was 50 years ago.

Roast Beef

FAT RELEASERS: beef, lettuce, tomato, onion, cheese, apple
- **Phase 2:** Order the Roast Beef with a Roast Chopped Farmhouse Salad without roast turkey, dressing, or bacon. Ask for a side of sliced apples.
- **Phase 3:** Reduce the beef by 1 ounce, or about 2 tablespoons, and add ½ bun.

Classic Turkey

FAT RELEASERS: turkey, lettuce, tomato, onion, cheese, apple, milk
- **Phase 2:** Get the Classic Turkey and a Roast Chopped Farmhouse Salad without roast turkey, dressing, or bacon. Ask for a side of sliced apples, and drink 1 bottle of Lowfat White Milk.
- **Phase 3:** Reduce the turkey by 1 ounce, or about 2 tablespoons, and add ½ bun.

Roast Chopped Farmhouse Salad

FAT RELEASERS: turkey, lettuce, tomato, onion, cheese, apple, milk

● **Phase 2:** Order the Roast Chopped Farmhouse Salad with no dressing or bacon, plus a side of sliced apples. To drink, get 1 bottle of Lowfat White Milk.

● **Phase 3:** Reduce the turkey by 1 ounce, or about 2 tablespoons, and add ½ bun.

Cravin' Chicken Sandwich

FAT RELEASERS: chicken, lettuce, tomato, onion, cheese, apple, milk

● **Phase 2:** Ask for the Roast Chicken Club Sandwich without the bacon, bun, or sauce and a Roast Chopped Farmhouse Salad without turkey, dressing, or bacon. Order sliced apples and 1 bottle of Lowfat White Milk.

● **Phase 3:** Reduce the chicken by 1 ounce, or about 2 tablespoons, and add ½ bun.

● WARNING! Fat Increaser Ahead

The traditional fast-food menu revolves around variations on meat and bread, whether the combo is a burger and bun, roast beef and a roll, or chicken in a wrap. Scan the entire menu, including descriptions of every dish, to uncover Digest Diet foods such as veggies, fat-free milk, and fruit.

AU BON PAIN

- Close to 250 cafés in 19 states across the United States
- (800) 825-5227; www.aubonpain.com

I love the extensive menu choices at Au Bon Pain, a chain that has a presence in malls, airports, colleges, and hospitals, in addition to freestanding restaurants. I recommend checking out the Hot & Cold Lunch Bar first—it has dozens of choices for putting together your meal. Another option—a favorite of mine—is to pair a cup of soup with a main dish. I eat half the main dish and refrigerate the rest for the next day. And Phase 1 diners, take note: we've called out several Au Bon Pain soup menu choices that are right for you!

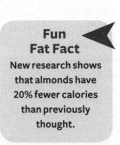

Fun Fat Fact
New research shows that almonds have 20% fewer calories than previously thought.

For nutrition information, you can look at a nutritional printout or build a virtual meal through a Café Smart Menu feature that lets you tinker with ingredients and see info on your choice of nutrients.

Southern Black-Eyed Pea Soup

FAT RELEASERS: celery, onion, carrot, ham, beans, chile pepper
- **Phase 1:** Order a large bowl (16 ounces) of Southern Black-Eyed Pea Soup.
- **Phases 2 and 3:** No change

12 Veggies Soup

FAT RELEASERS: tomato, squash, zucchini, carrot, onion, edamame, broccoli, leek, celery, mushrooms, corn
- **Phase 1:** Order the large bowl (16 ounces) of 12 Veggies Soup.
- **Phases 2 and 3:** No change

Black Bean Soup

FAT RELEASERS: black beans, garlic, onion
- **Phase 1:** Ask for a large bowl (16 ounces) of Black Bean Soup.
- **Phases 2 and 3:** No change

Carrot Ginger Soup

FAT RELEASERS: carrot, ginger, orange, honey
- **Phase 1:** Order the large bowl (16 ounces) of Carrot Ginger Soup.
- **Phases 2 and 3:** No change

French Moroccan Tomato Lentil Soup

FAT RELEASERS: tomato, lentils, beans, onion, garlic, chile peppers
- **Phase 1:** Ask for a large bowl (16 ounces) of French Moroccan Tomato Lentil Soup.
- **Phases 2 and 3:** No change

Garden Vegetable Soup

FAT RELEASERS: carrot, onion, celery, corn, bell pepper, zucchini, tomato, broccoli
- **Phase 1:** Ask for a large bowl (16 ounces) of Garden Vegetable Soup.
- **Phases 2 and 3:** No change

Gazpacho

FAT RELEASERS: tomato, cucumber, bell pepper
- **Phase 1:** Ask for a large bowl (16 ounces) of Gazpacho.
- **Phases 2 and 3:** No change

Roasted Eggplant Soup

FAT RELEASERS: eggplant, tomato, onion, cheese
- **Phase 1:** Ask for a large bowl (16 ounces) of Roasted Eggplant Soup.
- **Phases 2 and 3:** No change

Thai Coconut Curry Soup

FAT RELEASERS: ginger, coconut, potato, bell pepper, tomato, carrot, onion, spinach
- **Phase 1:** Ask for a large bowl (16 ounces) of Thai Coconut Curry Soup.
- **Phases 2 and 3:** No change

Tomato Cheddar Soup

FAT RELEASERS: tomato, garlic, cheese
- **Phase 1:** Ask for a large bowl (16 ounces) of Tomato Cheddar Soup.
- **Phases 2 and 3:** No change

Tuscan White Bean Soup

FAT RELEASERS: beans, tomato, onion, carrot, escarole, celery, leek, garlic, olive oil, chile pepper
- **Phase 1:** Order a large bowl (16 ounces) of Tuscan White Bean Soup.
- **Phases 2 and 3:** No change

Vegetarian Lentil Soup

FAT RELEASERS: lentils, onion, garlic, carrot, tomato
- **Phase 1:** Order a large bowl (16 ounces) of Vegetarian Lentil Soup.
- **Phases 2 and 3:** No change

Vegetarian Chili

FAT RELEASERS: beans, tomato, onion, bell pepper, carrot, garlic
- **Phase 1:** Ask for a large bowl (16 ounces) of Vegetarian Chili.
- **Phases 2 and 3:** No change

Beef Chili

FAT RELEASERS: beef, tomato, onion, beans, bell pepper, chile peppers, lime, lettuce, cucumber
- **Phase 2:** Ask for a medium bowl (12 ounces) of Beef Chili and a Garden Salad with no dressing or croutons.
- **Phase 3:** Reduce the chili to 1 cup and add ½ cup of rice.

WARNING! Fat Increaser Ahead

The ingredients and calories in restaurant chili range from reasonable to outrageous. Fatty cuts of beef and pork that are browned in oil, as well as fat increasing toppings like sour cream, pump up the calorie count in chili con carne. The smartest choice is vegetarian-style chili with a sprinkle of cheese on top.

Turkey Chili

FAT RELEASERS: turkey, beans, vegetables, tomato, lettuce, cucumber
- **Phase 2:** Order a medium bowl (12 ounces) of Turkey Chili and a Garden Salad with no dressing or croutons.
- **Phase 3:** Reduce the chili to 1 cup and add ½ cup of rice.

Chef's Salad

FAT RELEASERS: lettuce, turkey, ham, cheese, tomato, grapes
- **Phase 2:** Ask for a Chef's Salad with no dressing or bacon, plus 1 cup of fresh grapes.
- **Phase 3:** Reduce the turkey and ham by 1 ounce, or about 2 tablespoons. Add 1 slice of bread.

Mediterranean Chicken Salad

FAT RELEASERS: lettuce, chicken, cheese, tomato, olives, chickpeas, sesame seeds, cucumber
- **Phase 2:** Order the Mediterranean Chicken Salad without dressing and an order of Hummus and Cucumber.
- **Phase 3:** Reduce the chicken by 1 ounce, or about 2 tablespoons, and add 1 slice of bread.

Greek Salad

FAT RELEASERS: lettuce, tomato, cucumber, onion, artichoke, olives, cheese, chicken
- **Phase 2:** Order the Greek Salad with no dressing, plus 4 ounces of chicken breast.
- **Phase 3:** Reduce the cheese by 1 ounce, or about 2 tablespoons, and add 1 small roll.

Roast Beef

FAT RELEASERS: beef, carrot, tomato, cucumber
- **Phase 2:** Order 4 ounces of Roast Beef. For sides, ask for 1 cup of Roasted Carrots and 1 cup of Tomato Cucumber Salad.
- **Phase 3:** Reduce the beef by 1 ounce, or about 2 tablespoons. Add ½ cup of brown rice.

Ham

FAT RELEASERS: ham, green beans, almonds, pineapple
- **Phase 2:** Ask for 4 ounces of Ham with 1 cup of Roasted Green Beans with Almonds on the side and 1 cup of Fresh Pineapple.
- **Phase 3:** Order 3 ounces of Ham and add 1 small roll.

Chicken Breast

FAT RELEASERS: chicken, yogurt, cucumber, onion, watermelon, cheese

• **Phase 2:** From the lunch bar, get 4 ounces of Chicken Breast with 1 cup of Tsaziki and 1 cup of Watermelon and Feta Salad.

• **Phase 3:** Reduce the chicken by 1 ounce, or about 2 tablespoons, and add ½ pita.

Turkey Breast

FAT RELEASERS: turkey, lettuce, tomato, cucumber, artichoke, olives, cheese, onion, fruit

• **Phase 2:** Ask for 4 ounces of Turkey Breast with a Greek Salad without dressing and 1 small Fruit Cup.

• **Phase 3:** Reduce the turkey by 1 ounce, or about 2 tablespoons, and add ½ cup of quinoa.

Cheddar, Fruit, and Cracker Snack

FAT RELEASERS: cheese, fruit

• **All phases:** Have the Cheddar, Fruit, and Crackers without crackers.

Garden Salad Snack

FAT RELEASERS: lettuce, tomato, cucumber, nuts

• **All phases:** Order the Garden Salad without dressing or croutons and add ½ ounce of mixed nuts.

BAJA FRESH MEXICAN GRILL

● More than 400 locations
● (949) 270-8900; www.bajafresh.com

The Baja Fresh menu is easy to customize from the à la carte offerings. You can easily combine a protein—charbroiled steak or chicken, pork carnitas—with grilled or salad veggies for vitamin C and fiber, a dollop of guacamole for healthy fats, and beans to ramp up the fiber.

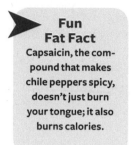

**Fun
Fat Fact**
Capsaicin, the compound that makes chile peppers spicy, doesn't just burn your tongue; it also burns calories.

When you order during Phase 2, be sure to specify that you don't want the rice, tortillas, or chips/strips that come standard with many orders. You can add a small corn tortilla or small scoop of rice for Phase 3 and take down the portion size of your protein. The website offers a Master Nutritional Table for checking out the numbers.

● **WARNING! Fat Increaser Ahead**
Tortillas and wraps are so skinny that it's hard to believe they're laden with calories. A 10-inch flour tortilla, which is barely large enough to wrap a burrito, has more than 200 calories. Tack on a couple of inches to fit the filling and calories rise almost to 300. Ordering your burrito bare or naked instantly removes a major fat increaser.

Baja Ensalada

FAT RELEASERS: beef, lettuce, tomato, onion, cheese
• **Phase 2:** Order a Baja Ensalada with tender steak.
• **Phase 3:** Reduce the steak by 1 ounce, or about 2 tablespoons, and add a 6-inch corn tortilla.

Baja Burrito Bare Style

FAT RELEASERS: chicken, bell pepper, chile peppers, onion, tomato, beans
• **Phase 2:** Ask for ½ order of Baja Burrito bare style with no rice. Order a side salad and verde sauce.
• **Phase 3:** Reduce the chicken by 1 ounce, or about 2 tablespoons, and add ½ cup of rice.

Baja Ensalada

FAT RELEASERS: chicken, lettuce, tomato, onion, cheese, avocado
• **Phase 2:** Ask for Baja Ensalada with fire-grilled chicken and a 3-ounce order of guacamole.
• **Phase 3:** Reduce the chicken by 1 ounce, or about 2 tablespoons. Add a 6-inch corn tortilla.

Fire-Grilled Chicken Tortilla Soup

FAT RELEASERS: chicken, tomato, avocado, cheese, onion, bell pepper, chile peppers
• **Phase 2:** Ask for Fire-Grilled Chicken Tortilla Soup and an order of Veggie Mix on the side.
• **Phase 3:** Reduce the chicken by 1 ounce, or about 2 tablespoons. Add ½ cup of rice.

Grilled Veggie Burrito Bare Style

FAT RELEASERS: bell pepper, chile peppers, onion, tomato, beans, cheese
• **Phase 2:** Order a Grilled Veggie Burrito bare style with no rice or sour cream.
• **Phase 3:** Reduce the beans by 1 ounce, or about 2 tablespoons. Add ½ cup of rice.

BENIHANA

- Close to 100 locations
- (800) 327-3369; www.benihana.com

Benihana specializes in a cooking method called *teppanyaki*—also referred to as *hibachi*—where your meal is cooked in front of you on an oversized griddle. When you order your meal, the first step is to go à la carte. Entrées routinely come with soup, salad, a grilled shrimp appetizer, vegetables, rice, and sauces. Needless to say, that's way too much food! Next, ask the chef to use less oil when cooking your meal. Finally, watch your portions and be prepared to bring home the extras. Nutrition info is not readily available, so use your best portion-estimating skills.

> **Fun Fat Fact**
> Spice up your meal with a side of pickled ginger. New research suggests that ginger increases post-meal calorie burning and enhances fullness.

> **WARNING! Fat Increaser Ahead**
> Digest Diet danger zones in traditional Japanese restaurants include oily stir-fries, fried tempura dishes, and big bowls of noodles. Instead, opt for fat releasers such as omega-3-rich fish, veggies with vitamin C, and the seasonings garlic and ginger.

Filet Mignon

FAT RELEASERS: beef, vegetables
• **Phase 2:** Ask for ½ order of Filet Mignon, plus an order of hibachi vegetables.
• **Phase 3:** Reduce the steak by 1 ounce, or about 2 tablespoons, and add ½ cup of brown rice.

Hibachi Steak

FAT RELEASERS: beef, mushrooms, vegetables
• **Phase 2:** Ask for ½ order of Hibachi Steak and an order of hibachi vegetables.
• **Phase 3:** Reduce the steak by 1 ounce, or about 2 tablespoons. Add ½ cup of brown rice.

Hibachi Chicken

FAT RELEASERS: chicken, mushrooms, sesame seeds, vegetables
• **Phase 2:** Ask for ½ order of Hibachi Chicken without butter and a side of hibachi vegetables.
• **Phase 3:** Reduce the chicken by 1 ounce, or about 2 tablespoons, and add ½ cup of brown rice.

Hibachi Lemon Chicken

FAT RELEASERS: chicken, mushrooms, lemon, vegetables
• **Phase 2:** Get ½ order of Hibachi Lemon Chicken without butter and a side of hibachi vegetables.
• **Phase 3:** Reduce the chicken by 1 ounce, or about 2 tablespoons, and add ½ cup of brown rice.

Emperor's Salad

FAT RELEASERS: chicken, lettuce, grapefruit, avocado, asparagus, cucumber, vegetables, vinegar
• **Phase 2:** Ask for ½ order of Emperor's Salad with chicken and no dressing or rice. On the side, get the Garden Delight without rice.
• **Phase 3:** Reduce the chicken by 1 ounce, or about 2 tablespoons, and add ½ cup of brown rice.

Hibachi Shrimp

FAT RELEASERS: shrimp, lettuce, vegetables
• **Phase 2:** Get ½ order of Hibachi Shrimp plus a green salad with no dressing and an order of hibachi vegetables.
• **Phase 3:** Reduce the shrimp by 1 ounce, or about 2 tablespoons. Add ½ cup of brown rice.

Hibachi Scallops

FAT RELEASERS: scallops, lemon, asparagus, vegetables, vinegar

● **Phase 2:** Ask for ½ order of Hibachi Scallops without butter. Order hibachi vegetables and the Garden Delight with no rice on the side.

● **Phase 3:** Reduce the scallops by 1 ounce, or about 2 tablespoons, and add ½ cup of brown rice.

Twin Lobster Tails

FAT RELEASERS: lobster, lemon, vegetables, asparagus, vinegar

● **Phase 2:** Ask for ½ order of Twin Lobster Tails with no butter. For sides, order hibachi vegetables and Garden Delight without rice.

● **Phase 3:** Reduce the lobster by 1 ounce, or about 2 tablespoons. Add ½ cup of brown rice.

Hibachi Tuna Steak

FAT RELEASERS: fish, tomato, avocado, edamame, sesame seeds, vinegar, vegetables

● **Phase 2:** Get ½ order of Hibachi Tuna Steak and hibachi vegetables on the side.

● **Phase 3:** Reduce the tuna by 1 ounce, or about 2 tablespoons, and add ½ cup of brown rice.

Sashimi

FAT RELEASERS: fish, asparagus, vegetables, vinegar

● **Phase 2:** Order 8 pieces of assorted Sashimi without rice. For sides, ask for Garden Delight without rice and hibachi vegetables.

● **Phase 3:** Reduce the fish to 6 pieces and add ½ cup of brown rice.

BOB EVANS

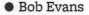

- 600 restaurants in 18 states
- (800) 939-2338; www.bobevans.com

Bob Evans offers traditional American casual dining fare, including all-day breakfasts, burgers, and family-style dishes. The chain also promotes health and nutrition through a dedicated page on its website and healthful dishes that are highlighted on the menu. As with most restaurants serving American cuisine, Bob Evans has a few items that you can order and eat as is and others that you'll have to request à la carte, such as the meat from a sandwich or the entrée from a dinner. Remember to speak up with basic requests to leave off salad dressing and fat increaser ingredients like bacon, dried cranberries (they're dunked in sugar syrup before drying), and candied pecans. To do your homework ahead of time, visit the nutrition info page on the restaurant website.

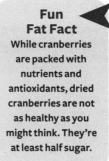

Fun Fat Fact

While cranberries are packed with nutrients and antioxidants, dried cranberries are not as healthy as you might think. They're at least half sugar.

Heritage Chef Salad

FAT RELEASERS: turkey, ham, cheese, egg, lettuce, tomato, scallions
● **Phase 2:** Order the Savor size Heritage Chef Salad without bacon or dressing.
● **Phase 3:** Reduce the turkey and ham by 1 ounce, or about 2 tablespoons, and add 1 slice of wheat bread.

Apple Cranberry Spinach Salad

FAT RELEASERS: chicken, spinach, apple, beans
● **Phase 2:** Ask for the Apple Cranberry Spinach Salad without cranberries, pecans, or dressing. On the side, get an order of Farm Festival Bean Soup.
● **Phase 3:** Reduce the chicken by 1 ounce, or about 2 tablespoons, and add 1 slice of wheat bread.

Roast Beef

FAT RELEASERS: beef, broccoli, lettuce, vegetables, milk
● **Phase 2:** Ask for 4 ounces of Roast Beef, plus Fresh Steamed Broccoli and a Farmhouse Garden Salad without dressing or croutons. Also, order a regular size 2% white milk.
● **Phase 3:** Reduce the beef by 1 ounce, or about 2 tablespoons. Add 1 slice of wheat bread.

Grilled Chicken

FAT RELEASERS: chicken, broccoli, beef, vegetables, lettuce, fruit, milk
● **Phase 2:** Order the Grilled Chicken entrée, Hearty Beef Vegetable Soup, a Farmhouse Garden Salad without dressing or croutons, fresh fruit plate, and Original Cappuccino.
● **Phase 3:** Reduce the chicken by 1 ounce, or about 2 tablespoons. Add ½ plain baked potato.

Grilled Salmon Fillet

FAT RELEASERS: salmon, broccoli, lettuce, vegetables, fruit
● **Phase 2:** Ask for the Salmon Fillet entrée with no potato, plus Fresh Steamed Broccoli, Farmhouse Garden Salad without dressing or croutons, and a fresh fruit plate.
● **Phase 3:** Reduce the salmon by 1 ounce, or about 2 tablespoons, and add ½ plain baked potato.

Veggie Omelet

FAT RELEASERS: egg, spinach, onion, tomato, fruit, milk
● **Phase 2:** Order the Veggie Omelet made with real eggs and skip the toast. Instead, have 1 fresh fruit plate and an Original Cappuccino.
● **Phase 3:** Order 1 egg scrambled with vegetables and add 1 slice of plain wheat toast.

BOSTON MARKET

- 490 restaurants nationwide
- (800) 877-2870; www.bostonmarket.com

You can find plenty to eat on the Boston Market menu, although not always in Digest Diet portions. The chain is known for its chicken, and there's no need to order skinless—just remove the skin before eating. Choose vegetables (hot or cold) that don't look like they're swimming in fat. Boston Market doesn't have whole-grain options for Phase 3, so enjoy a small portion of one of the available grains or potato dishes we suggest (or one item from the Whole Grains To Go Kit on page 10). The website offers frequently updated nutrition information through its food page.

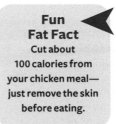

Fun Fat Fact
Cut about 100 calories from your chicken meal— just remove the skin before eating.

● **WARNING! Fat Increaser Ahead**
Always order Caesar and other salads without dressing and fat increaser toppings. Caesar salad, which is said to have been invented in Mexico in the 1920s, traditionally contains Parmesan cheese and high-calorie croutons and is drenched with an oily dressing.

Beef Brisket

FAT RELEASERS: beef, broccoli, carrot, squash, green beans
• **Phase 2:** Order a regular (4-ounce) Beef Brisket, plus Fresh Steamed Vegetables and Green Beans.
• **Phase 3:** Reduce the beef by 1 ounce, or about 2 tablespoons, and add ½ cup of Garlic Dill New Potatoes.

Rotisserie Chicken ¼ White

FAT RELEASERS: chicken, lettuce, cheese, broccoli, carrot, squash, green beans
• **Phase 2:** Ask for the Rotisserie Chicken ¼ White (remove the skin before eating); plus a Caesar Salad with no croutons, chicken, or dressing; and 1 order of Fresh Steamed Vegetables.
• **Phase 3:** Reduce the chicken by 1 ounce, or about 2 tablespoons, and add ½ cup, or about ½ order, of Rice Pilaf.

Rotisserie Chicken Dark

FAT RELEASERS: chicken, tomato, chile peppers, onion, green beans
• **Phase 2:** Order 1 thigh and 1 drumstick of Rotisserie Chicken Dark and remove the skin before eating. For sides, ask for an order of Tortilla Soup without toppings and an order of Green Beans.
• **Phase 3:** Reduce the chicken by 1 ounce, or about 2 tablespoons. Add 1 small piece of Cornbread.

Turkey Breast

FAT RELEASERS: turkey, lettuce, cheese, broccoli, carrot, squash, green beans
• **Phase 2:** Ask for the regular (5-ounce) Turkey Breast with a Caesar Salad with no croutons, chicken, or dressing; and an order of Fresh Steamed Vegetables.
• **Phase 3:** Reduce the turkey by 1 ounce, or about 2 tablespoons, and add ½ cup, or about ½ order, of Rice Pilaf.

Mediterranean Salad

FAT RELEASERS: lettuce, chicken, cucumbers, tomato, cheese
• **Phase 2:** Ask for ½ order of the Mediterranean Salad without dressing or chips, plus 1 piece of Rotisserie Chicken Dark, removing the skin before eating.
• **Phase 3:** Reduce the chicken by 1 ounce, or about 2 tablespoons, and add ½ cup, about ½ order, of Garlic Dill New Potatoes.

Southwest Santa Fe Salad

FAT RELEASERS: lettuce, beans, chicken, cheese, tomato, onion
• **Phase 2:** Ask for ½ order of the Southwest Santa Fe Salad without dressing or tortilla strips. Order a side of Green Beans.
• **Phase 3:** Reduce the chicken by 1 ounce, or about 2 tablespoons. Add 1 small piece of cornbread.

BUBBA GUMP SHRIMP CO.

- About 36 locations nationwide and internationally
- (800) 552-6379; www.bubbagump.com

As its name suggests, Bubba Gump is known for its shrimp, although the menu also offers seafood, fish, chicken, and steak. Vegetables are somewhat lacking—your only options are green salad, the "Spring Mix" topping for sandwiches, veggies cooked on a skewer, and the veggies in a "skillet" meal. So ask the waitstaff if you can put together your own combination of protein plus vegetables. No whole grains here; you get to pick between rice and mashed potatoes in Phase 3 (or bring an item from the Whole Grains To Go Kit on page 10). Nutrition info is not readily available. To check out calories, go to the website and choose a location in New York City or another city that requires the posting of calorie information. Then click on the menu.

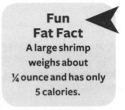

Fun Fat Fact
A large shrimp weighs about ¼ ounce and has only 5 calories.

● WARNING! Fat Increaser Ahead

Frying foods generally adds at least a tablespoon of fat, depending on the type and amount of breading, the temperature of the oil, and how well the food is drained. The difference between a 4-ounce portion of steamed shrimp and the same amount of fried shrimp is about 200 calories, mostly from oil.

Certified Angus Top Sirloin

FAT RELEASERS: beef, vegetables
- **Phase 2:** Get ½ order (5 ounces) of Certified Angus Top Sirloin with no onions or potatoes. For a side, ask for skillet vegetables.
- **Phase 3:** Reduce the steak by 1 ounce, or about 2 tablespoons, and add ½ cup, about ½ order, of mashed potatoes.

Classic Caesar Salad with Grilled Chicken

FAT RELEASERS: lettuce, chicken, shrimp, tomato
- **Phase 2:** Order the Classic Caesar Salad with Grilled Chicken without dressing or croutons, plus a Traditional Shrimp Cocktail with Horseradish.
- **Phase 3:** Reduce the chicken by 1 ounce, or about 2 tablespoons, and add ½ bun.

Shrimpin' Dippin' Broth

FAT RELEASERS: shrimp, lettuce, chicken
- **Phase 2:** Order the Shrimpin' Dippin' Broth, and skip the rice and bread. Order the Classic Caesar Salad with Grilled Chicken without dressing or croutons.
- **Phase 3:** Reduce the chicken by 1 ounce, or about 2 tablespoons, and add ½ cup, about ½ order, of rice.

Shrimp Chimichurri Skewers

FAT RELEASERS: shrimp, bell pepper, onion, squash, vegetables, lettuce
- **Phase 2:** Ask for the Shrimp Chimichurri Skewers without rice or sauce, plus 1 order of skewer vegetables and 1 of Spring Mix.
- **Phase 3:** Reduce the shrimp by 2 shrimp. Add ½ cup, about ½ order, of rice.

Shrimp & Veggie Skewers

FAT RELEASERS: shrimp, bell pepper, red onion, squash
- **Phase 2:** Ask for 2 orders of Shrimp & Veggie Skewers.
- **Phase 3:** Reduce the shrimp by 2 shrimp, and add ½ cup, about ½ order, of rice.

Shrimper's Net Catch

FAT RELEASERS: shrimp, lettuce, vegetables
- **Phase 2:** Ask for ½ order of Shrimper's Net Catch plus an order of Spring Mix without dressing and an order of skillet vegetables.
- **Phase 3:** Reduce the shrimp by 1 ounce, or about 2 tablespoons, and add ½ cup, about ½ order, of mashed potatoes.

Steamed Crab Legs

FAT RELEASERS: crab, vegetables
● **Phase 2:** Ask for ½ order of Steamed Crab Legs, and skip the butter, rice, and coleslaw. Order Skewer Vegetables on the side.
● **Phase 3:** Add 1 small roll.

Salmon & Veggie Skillet

FAT RELEASERS: salmon, vegetables
● **Phase 2:** Order the Salmon & Veggie Skillet without rice.
● **Phase 3:** Reduce the salmon by 1 ounce, or about 2 tablespoons, and add ½ cup of rice.

WARNING! Fat Increaser Ahead

A restaurant meal almost never has the right balance of veggies, protein, and grains. That's why it's so important to get used to eating about the same types and amounts of foods each day. When you go to a restaurant, you'll know exactly what to order.

BURGER KING

- More than 12,400 worldwide
- (866) 394-2493; www.bk.com

Most fast-food burger places, Burger King included,

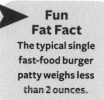

Fun Fat Fact

The typical single fast-food burger patty weighs less than 2 ounces.

offer varying combinations of burgers, salads, and fruit (usually apples). There's not a lot of room to be creative with your meal! And even the largest salad may fall short of our recommended 2 cups. Burger King's full nutrition chart is available on the website.

Hamburger Patty

FAT RELEASERS: beef, lettuce, tomato, cheese, apple, milk
- **Phase 2:** Ask for a plain hamburger patty and 1 Garden Side Salad without dressing or croutons plus BK Fresh Apple Slices. To drink, ask for an 8-ounce fat-free milk.
- **Phase 3:** Add ½ bun.

Tendergrill Chicken

FAT RELEASERS: chicken, lettuce, tomato, cheese, apple, milk,
- **Phase 2:** Ask for 1 Tendergrill Chicken patty with 1 Garden Side Salad without dressing or croutons and BK Fresh Apple Slices. To drink, ask for an 8-ounce fat-free milk.
- **Phase 3:** Add ½ bun.

Chicken Caesar Garden Fresh Salad

FAT RELEASERS: chicken, lettuce, tomato, cheese, apple, milk

● **Phase 2:** Order the Chicken Caesar Garden Fresh Salad without dressing or croutons, plus BK Fresh Apple Slices, and an 8-ounce fat-free milk.

● **Phase 3:** Reduce the chicken by 1 ounce, or about 2 tablespoons. Add ½ bun.

Chicken, Apple, and Cranberry Garden Fresh Salad

FAT RELEASERS: chicken, lettuce, apple, cheese, milk

● **Phase 2:** Ask for the Chicken, Apple, and Cranberry Garden Fresh Salad, and skip the dressing and cranberries. Add BK Fresh Apple Slices and an 8-ounce fat-free milk.

● **Phase 3:** Reduce the chicken by 1 ounce, or about 2 tablespoons, and add ½ bun.

● WARNING! Fat Increaser Ahead

Although fast-food menus have improved greatly over the past few years, they're still filled with fat increasers like buns made with refined flour, fatty fried foods, and sugary drinks. You'll have to tease out the good stuff by looking for grilled protein, fresh vegetables, fat-free milk, and fruit.

CARL'S JR.

● More than 1,100 restaurants in 14 states
● (877) 799-7827; www.carlsjr.com

> **Fun Fat Fact**
>
> Some say that it takes more calories to digest lettuce than the lettuce provides. While it's not true, it's pretty close. A cup of lettuce has only 5 or so calories.

Although extremely limited in Digest Diet fare, the menu at Carl's Jr. does offer a few less common fast-food fat releasers, such as pineapple, green chili peppers, and buns with whole wheat. Mix and match is the rule of the day. The Carl's Jr. nutrition calculator on the website allows you to view full nutrition info on menu items, but you can't customize your meal online.

Beef Patty

FAT RELEASERS: beef, lettuce, carrot, cabbage, tomato, onion, cheese, avocado
● **Phase 2:** Ask for 1 beef patty, plus 1 side salad without dressing or croutons, an order of lettuce, tomato, and red onion, 1 slice of Swiss cheese, and 1 scoop of guacamole.
● **Phase 3:** Eliminate the cheese and add ½ honey wheat bun.

Turkey Patty

FAT RELEASERS: turkey, pineapple, lettuce, carrot, cabbage, cheese, chile pepper
● **Phase 2:** Order 1 turkey patty with an order of pineapple slices, a side salad without dressing or croutons, 1 scoop of green chili peppers, and 1 scoop of shredded cheddar/jack cheese.
● **Phase 3:** Eliminate the cheese and add ½ honey wheat bun.

WARNING! Fat Increaser Ahead

Turkey burger patties may contain as much fat and calories as a beef patty. The juiciest turkey burgers also tend to have the most calories, as they often contain dark meat turkey plus added skin for moisture and flavor. A quick check of calorie counts on a restaurant website will show whether switching to turkey makes much difference.

Chicken Breast

FAT RELEASERS: chicken, lettuce, carrot, cabbage, cheese, avocado, pineapple
• **Phase 2:** Ask for 1 chicken breast, a side salad without dressing or croutons, 1 scoop of guacamole, and 1 order of pineapple slices.
• **Phase 3:** Reduce the chicken by 1 ounce, or about 2 tablespoons, and add ½ honey wheat bun.

Cranberry Apple Walnut Chicken Salad

FAT RELEASERS: chicken, lettuce, carrot, cabbage, cheese, apple, avocado
• **Phase 2:** Order the Cranberry Apple Walnut Chicken Salad, but skip the dressing, walnuts, and cranberries. Ask for 1 scoop of guacamole.
• **Phase 3:** Reduce the chicken by 1 ounce, or about 2 tablespoons. Add ½ honey wheat bun.

Original Grilled Chicken Salad

FAT RELEASERS: chicken, lettuce, carrot, cabbage, cheese, onion, cucumber, tomato
• **Phase 2:** Ask for the Original Grilled Chicken Salad without dressing or croutons, plus an extra chicken breast.
• **Phase 3:** Reduce the chicken by 1 ounce, or about 2 tablespoons. Add ½ honey wheat bun.

THE CHEESECAKE FACTORY

- Close to 170 locations across the country
- (818) 871-3000; www.thecheesecakefactory.com

The Cheesecake Factory menu is huge and so are its portions. The chain is not very forthcoming with nutrition information so you'll have to trust us when we tell you that portions served are at least twice as large as we recommend. To the chain's credit, the menu now includes Skinnylicious meals, although you'll still need to customize them. But there's plenty to choose from, as The Cheesecake Factory has more vegetable options and dishes with vegetables on its menu than almost any other chain. We couldn't find whole grains on the menu; the restaurant you go to might be different as menu choices change somewhat from city to city.

> **Fun Fat Fact**
>
> It's all good when you're eating fish. Most with white-colored flesh are low in fat and calories, while darker fish like tuna and salmon are packed with omega-3s.

> **WARNING! Fat Increaser Ahead**
>
> Restaurant menus often are filled with fat- and sugar-rich desserts and other foods that are hard to resist. But research shows that the more you say no to temptation, the stronger your willpower becomes. So reach for fruit when the urge strikes.

Factory Chopped Salad

FAT RELEASERS: lettuce, chicken, tomato, avocado, cheese, apple, beef
- **Phase 2:** Ask for ½ order of Factory Chopped Salad, but skip the bacon, corn, and vinaigrette. Add 1 charbroiled burger patty.
- **Phase 3:** Eliminate the avocado, and add ½ plain baked potato.

Greek Salad

FAT RELEASERS: lettuce, tomato, cucumber, onion, olives, arugula, chicken
- **Phase 2:** Ask for ½ order of Greek Salad without vinaigrette, plus 4 ounces of grilled chicken breast.
- **Phase 3:** Reduce the chicken by 1 ounce, or about 2 tablespoons, and add 1 slice of bread.

Chinese Chicken Salad

FAT RELEASERS: lettuce, chicken, scallions, almonds, bean sprouts, orange, sesame seeds
- **Phase 2:** Get ½ order of Chinese Chicken Salad with no noodles, wontons, or dressing.
- **Phase 3:** Reduce the chicken by 1 ounce, or about 2 tablespoons. Add 1 slice of bread.

Luau Salad

FAT RELEASERS: lettuce, chicken, cucumber, scallions, bell pepper, green beans, carrot, mango, sesame seeds
- **Phase 2:** Ask for a ½ order of Luau Salad without wontons, macadamia nuts, or dressing.
- **Phase 3:** Reduce the chicken by 1 ounce, or about 2 tablespoons, and add ½ cup of rice.

Chargrilled Coulotte Steak

FAT RELEASERS: beef, lettuce, vegetables, asparagus
- **Phase 2:** Ask for ½ order (5 ounces) of Chargrilled Coulotte Steak, no butter, plus a side salad without dressing and 1 order of asparagus.
- **Phase 3:** Reduce the steak by 1 ounce, or about 2 tablespoons, and add ½ cup, about ½ order, of Santorini Farro Salad.

Roadside Sliders

FAT RELEASERS: beef, kale, green beans, apple, almonds
- **Phase 2:** Order 2 Roadside Sliders without buns, plus a Fresh Kale Salad without cranberries or dressing.
- **Phase 3:** Decrease to 1 Roadside Slider and add 1 slice of bread.

Salisbury Chopped Steak

FAT RELEASERS: beef, onion, mushrooms, garlic, lettuce, asparagus, beets, cheese

• **Phase 2:** Ask for ½ order of Salisbury Chopped Steak, plus ½ order of French Country Salad without pecans or vinaigrette.

• **Phase 3:** Reduce the steak by 1 ounce, or about 2 tablespoons, and add ½ cup, about ½ order, of mashed potatoes.

Baja Chicken Tacos

FAT RELEASERS: chicken, avocado, tomato, onion, cilantro, black beans

• **Phase 2:** Get ½ order of Baja Chicken Tacos without tortillas, crema, or rice.

• **Phase 3:** Reduce the chicken by 1 ounce, or about 2 tablespoons, and add ½ cup of rice.

Lemon-Herb Roasted Chicken

FAT RELEASERS: chicken, lemon, herbs, lettuce, cheese, avocado, pear, orange

• **Phase 2:** Ask for ½ order of Lemon-Herb Roasted Chicken without potatoes or sauce, and remove the skin. On the side, order ½ Carlton Salad without vinaigrette, chicken, cranberries, or raisins.

• **Phase 3:** Reduce the chicken by 1 ounce, or about 2 tablespoons. Add ½ cup of potatoes.

Grilled Turkey Patty

FAT RELEASERS: turkey, mushrooms, garlic, lettuce, egg, cheese

• **Phase 2:** Order 1 grilled turkey patty, plus ½ order of Boston House Salad with no bacon, croutons, or dressing.

• **Phase 3:** Eliminate the cheese from the salad and add the skinnier half of the bun.

Ahi Tartare

FAT RELEASERS: tuna, avocado, ginger, sesame seeds, endive, radicchio, cheese

• **Phase 2:** Get ½ order of Ahi Tartare and ½ order of endive salad with no pecans or vinaigrette.

• **Phase 3:** Reduce the tuna by 1 ounce, or about 2 tablespoons, and add ½ cup of rice.

Fresh Grilled Salmon

FAT RELEASERS: salmon, vegetables, asparagus, green beans, tomato, cucumber, beets, apple, soybeans, radicchio, lettuce, cheese

• **Phase 2:** Get ½ order of Fresh Grilled Salmon, plus ½ order of Fresh Vegetable Salad without vinaigrette or chicken.

• **Phase 3:** Reduce the salmon by 1 ounce, and add ½ plain baked potato.

CHICK-FIL-A

- More than 1,615 locations in 39 states and Washington, D.C.
- (404) 765-8038; www.chick-fil-a.com

Chick-Fil-A has lots of fans of its grilled chicken, variety of salad veggies, and fruit salad (yay for resveratrol in the red grapes!). We came up with several different meals, although we had to bump up the protein by adding a half order of extra chicken. Unfortunately, this means you'll need to buy two meals to have one; bring home the other half for a later meal.

For Phase 3, we were happy to see multigrain bread! You can access nutrition information dish-by-dish or put together a few items using a meal calculator.

Fun Fat Fact

Sunflower seeds deliver fat releasing healthy fats, along with several minerals that you need for overall health, including copper, manganese, selenium, and phosphorus.

● WARNING! Fat Increaser Ahead

Figuring out the right portion of flatbread or pita can be challenging. The ideal size is no bigger than a 6-inch corn tortilla (about the size of a saucer) but most are larger. Some restaurants brush their breads with oil before or after baking, adding extra fat and calories.

Chargrilled Chicken Cool Wrap

FAT RELEASERS: chicken, lettuce, cabbage, carrot, tomato, cheese, broccoli, strawberries, grapes, apple, orange

• **Phase 2:** Order the Chargrilled Chicken Cool Wrap without flatbread or dressing. Add ½ order of chargrilled chicken breast, a side salad without croutons or dressing, and a fruit cup.

• **Phase 3:** Reduce the chicken by 1 ounce, or about 2 tablespoons, and add ½ multigrain flatbread.

Chargrilled & Fruit Salad

FAT RELEASERS: chicken, lettuce, cabbage, carrot, cheese, strawberries, grapes, apple, orange

• **Phase 2:** Ask for the Chargrilled & Fruit Salad without dressing, plus ½ order of chargrilled chicken breast and a fruit cup.

• **Phase 3:** Reduce the chicken by 1 ounce, or about 2 tablespoons, and add ½ multigrain flatbread.

Chargrilled Chicken Garden Salad

FAT RELEASERS: chicken, lettuce, cabbage, carrot, tomato, broccoli, cheese, sunflower seeds, honey, strawberries, grapes, apple, orange

• **Phase 2:** Order the Chargrilled Chicken Garden Salad without croutons or dressing, plus ½ chargrilled chicken breast and a fruit cup.

• **Phase 3:** Reduce the chicken by 1 ounce, or about 2 tablespoons, and add ½ multigrain flatbread.

Southwest Chargrilled Salad

FAT RELEASERS: chicken, lettuce, cabbage, carrot, tomato, corn, black beans, cheese, strawberries, grapes, apple, orange

• **Phase 2:** Ask for the Southwest Chargrilled Salad, but skip the tortilla strips and dressing. Add ½ chargrilled chicken breast and a fruit cup.

• **Phase 3:** Reduce the chicken by 1 ounce, or about 2 tablespoons, and add ½ multigrain flatbread.

CHILI'S

- 1,282 locations nationwide
- (800) 983-4637; www.chilis.com

Chili's offers a lot of dishes inspired by Mexican cuisine, which is rich in fat releasers such as MUFA-rich avocado and resveratrol-rich red wine. You definitely need to put together your meal with à la carte items—the salmon from a salmon dinner, grilled chicken without the accompanying side dishes, steamed broccoli from the side dish list—rather than ordering from the full meal options that have as many fat increasers as releasers. Also, ask for oil and butter to be left off your order; if they're already a part of the dish, request other options with fewer fat increasers.

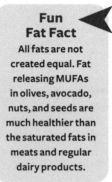

Fun Fat Fact

All fats are not created equal. Fat releasing MUFAs in olives, avocado, nuts, and seeds are much healthier than the saturated fats in meats and regular dairy products.

WARNING! Fat Increaser Ahead

When you order fajitas, stick with the protein plus veggies and salsa. The tortillas, sour cream, and cheese that come with your order can double or even triple the calories in your meal.

Classic Sirloin

FAT RELEASERS: beef, broccoli, lettuce, tomato, onion, cucumber, cheese
- **Phase 2:** Ask for the Classic Sirloin entrée order, plus a House Salad with no croutons or dressing.
- **Phase 3:** Reduce the beef by 1 ounce, or about 2 tablespoons. Add ½ cup of rice.

Chicken Fajitas

FAT RELEASERS: chicken, bell pepper, onion, red wine
- **Phase 2:** Order the Chicken Fajitas, but skip the tortillas and condiments. Have a 4-ounce glass of red wine on the side.
- **Phase 3:** Reduce the chicken by 1 ounce, or about 2 tablespoons, and add ½ cup, about ½ order, of rice.

Margarita Grilled Chicken

FAT RELEASERS: chicken, lettuce, tomato, onion, cucumber, cheese, vinegar, red wine
- **Phase 2:** Order the Margarita Grilled Chicken without side dishes, plus a House Salad without dressing or croutons and with vinegar. Have 4 ounces of red wine.
- **Phase 3:** Reduce the chicken by 1 ounce, or about 2 tablespoons, and add ½ cup, about ½ order, of rice.

Grilled Salmon with Garlic and Herbs

FAT RELEASERS: salmon, lettuce, tomato, onion, cucumber, cheese, vinegar
- **Phase 2:** Ask for 1 order of Grilled Salmon with Garlic and Herbs, no sides, and a House Salad without dressing or croutons and with vinegar.
- **Phase 3:** Reduce the salmon by 1 ounce, or about 2 tablespoons, and add ½ cup, about ½ order, of rice.

Terlingua Chili

FAT RELEASERS: beans, tomato, onion, cheese, avocado
- **Phase 2:** Order a bowl of Terlingua Chili with toppings and an order of avocado slices.
- **Phase 3:** Eliminate the avocado, and add a 6-inch corn tortilla.

CHIPOTLE

- More than 300 locations nationwide
- (303) 595-4000; www.chipotle.com

At Chipotle, dishes are prepared to your specification so you can load up on more fat releasers and easily avoid fat increasers. Their website offers detailed nutritional information for each ingredient, if you're interested, and the servers at each restaurant tend to be friendly and well informed.

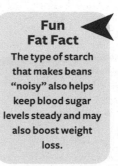

Fun Fat Fact

The type of starch that makes beans "noisy" also helps keep blood sugar levels steady and may also boost weight loss.

In Phase 2, your best choices are salads that you can craft from fat releasers like vegetables (full of fiber and vitamin C) and beans, topped with salsa made with more fresh veggies and fat releaser seasonings. All of their protein choices are served in reasonable portion sizes and prepared with minimal fat, so they are excellent fat releasers. In Phase 3, you can add rice or a tortilla.

WARNING! Fat Increaser Ahead

Portion size always is important, even for foods that are fat releasers. Consider the avocado, a nutrition-packed healthy fat. A quarter of an avocado has about 80 calories. If you were to eat a half instead, over one-third of your meal calories would be contributed from the avocado.

Fajitas

FAT RELEASERS: beef, bell pepper, onion, chile pepper, corn, beans
- **Phase 2:** Make fajitas with an order of steak (chicken or beans work, too), an order of fajita vegetables, an order of Roasted Chili-Corn Salsa, and an order of pinto beans.
- **Phase 3:** Reduce the steak by 1 ounce, or about 2 tablespoons, and add 1 soft corn tortilla.

Chicken Salad

FAT RELEASERS: lettuce, beans, cheese, chicken
- **Phase 2:** Make a chicken salad with 1 salad portion of romaine lettuce, an order of black beans, an order of cheese, and an order of chicken.
- **Phase 3:** Reduce the chicken by 1 ounce, or about 2 tablespoons, and add 1 soft corn tortilla.

Guacamole Salad

FAT RELEASERS: lettuce, avocado, bell pepper, onion, beans, cheese, tomato
- **Phase 2:** Make your own guacamole salad with 1 salad portion of romaine lettuce, an order of guacamole, an order of fajita vegetables, an order of black beans, an order of cheese, and an order of fresh tomato salsa.
- **Phase 3:** Reduce the guacamole by 1 ounce, or about 2 tablespoons, and add 1 soft corn tortilla.

CHUCK E. CHEESE'S

● More than 500 entertainment centers
● (888) 778-7193; www.chuckecheese.com

Wisely, Chuck E. Cheese's has some grown-up fare on its kid-centric menu. But nothing quite fit the Digest Diet guidelines, so we had to create our own meals. The Vegetarian Pizza is a nice treat for Phase 3.

> ### Fun Fat Fact
> The cheese served in restaurants almost always is full fat, so figure about 50 calories per thin slice and 25 calories per tablespoon shredded.

Roasted Chicken Salad

FAT RELEASERS: chicken, cheese, lettuce, tomato, vegetables, orange
● **Phase 2:** Make a roasted chicken salad with roasted chicken and cheese from the Roasted Chicken Ciabatta, plus 2 cups of fresh veggies from the Garden Fresh Salad Bar. Add ½ cup (1 side order) of mandarin oranges.
● **Phase 3:** Reduce the chicken by 1 ounce, or about 2 tablespoons, and add ½ ciabatta roll.

Vegetarian Pizza

FAT RELEASERS: cheese, onion, bell pepper, mushrooms, tomato, black olives, carrot, fruit
● **Phase 3:** Have 1 medium slice of Vegetarian Pizza, plus 1 cup of the Veggie Platter with no dressing, and ask for ¼ cup (1 ounce) of provolone cheese, 1 order of carrot sticks, and an order of Side Fruit Garnish.

COSI

● More than 100 restaurants in 16 states and the District of Columbia
● (847) 597-8800; www.getcosi.com

Between its standard salads and the dozens of items used in sandwiches and salads, Cosi offers lots of opportunity to create your own Digest Diet meals. Our biggest complaint is that the protein portions are small, so we had to add extra protein to meet our nutritional guidelines. Just ask for a double portion, though be warned you may be charged extra for this. The whole-grain flatbread is delicious but high in calories, so just eat half. Nutrition information is available item by item through the nutrition tab on the website.

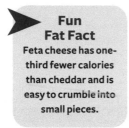

Fun Fat Fact

Feta cheese has one-third fewer calories than cheddar and is easy to crumble into small pieces.

Moroccan Lentil Soup

FAT RELEASERS: lentils
● **Phase 1:** Ask for a large (16-ounce) Moroccan Lentil Soup.
● **Phases 2 and 3:** No change

Signature Salad

FAT RELEASERS: lettuce, cheese, grapes, pear, pistachios, chicken
● **Phase 2:** Order the Signature Salad without dressing, cranberries, or bread, and add an extra order of chicken.
● **Phase 3:** Reduce the chicken by 1 ounce, or about 2 tablespoons, and add ½ piece of whole-grain flatbread.

Tandoori Chicken Salad

FAT RELEASERS: chicken, lettuce, bell pepper, tomato, onion, fruit
• **Phase 2:** Order the Tandoori Chicken Salad, but skip the dressing and ask for an extra order of chicken. Also have 1 cup of fruit salad.
• **Phase 3:** Reduce the chicken by 1 ounce, or about 2 tablespoons, and add ½ piece of whole-grain flatbread.

Shanghai Chicken Salad

FAT RELEASERS: lettuce, carrot, scallions, chicken, fruit
• **Phase 2:** Ask for the Shanghai Chicken Salad with no dressing or noodles, plus an extra order of chicken and 1 cup of fruit salad.
• **Phase 3:** Reduce the chicken by 1 ounce, or about 2 tablespoons, and add ½ piece of whole-grain flatbread.

Grilled Chicken Caesar Salad

FAT RELEASERS: chicken, lettuce, cheese, fruit
• **Phase 2:** Ask for the Grilled Chicken Caesar Salad without dressing or croutons. Add an extra order of chicken and 1 cup of fruit salad on the side.
• **Phase 3:** Reduce the chicken by 1 ounce, or about 2 tablespoons, and add ½ piece of whole-grain flatbread.

WARNING!
Fat Increaser Ahead

A standard "cup" or packet holds 2 ounces or 4 tablespoons of salad dressing and up to about 300 calories. The sugar and starches in fat-free dressings make them an unsuitable alternative. Your best bet is to sprinkle your salad with vinegar and add a few dashes of olive oil.

Asian Salmon Salad

FAT RELEASERS: salmon, lettuce, pineapple, carrots, edamame, red peppers, fruit
• **Phase 2:** Order the Wild Alaskan Salmon Salad without dressing, and 1 cup of fruit salad.
• **Phase 3:** Reduce the salmon by 1 ounce, or about 2 tablespoons. Add ½ piece of whole-grain flatbread.

Greek Salad

FAT RELEASERS: lettuce, tomato, cucumber, onion, cheese, olives, fruit
• **Phase 2:** Ask for the Greek Salad without dressing or bread. Add an extra order of feta cheese and 1 cup of fruit salad.
• **Phase 3:** Reduce the cheese by 1 ounce, or about 2 tablespoons, and add ½ piece of whole-grain flatbread.

CRACKER BARREL

- More than 600 in 42 states
- (800) 333-9566; www.crackerbarrel.com

Cracker Barrel features standard "hearty" American fare with little opportunity for customized prep. Although we know that the beans and carrots are prepared with fat, we recommend them over not having veggies at all. You'll notice by our Phase 3 recommendations that Cracker Barrel may not have whole-grain options so, you may want to pull out your Whole Grains To Go Kit (see page 10) here.

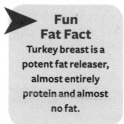

Fun Fat Fact
Turkey breast is a potent fat releaser, almost entirely protein and almost no fat.

Half Pound Hamburger

FAT RELEASERS: beef, lettuce, tomato, onion, green beans
- **Phase 2:** Ask for ½ order of the Half Pound Hamburger with no bun or fixings. On the side, have a tossed salad without dressing and an order of Country Green Beans.
- **Phase 3:** No change

Grilled Sirloin Steak

FAT RELEASERS: beef, green beans, carrot
- **Phase 2:** Have ½ order (4 ounces) of the Grilled Sirloin Steak, meat only. For sides, get Country Green Beans and Sweet Whole Baby Carrots.
- **Phase 3:** Reduce the beef by 1 ounce, or about 2 tablespoons. Add ½ cup of Mashed Potatoes.

Open-Faced Roast Beef

FAT RELEASERS: beef, lettuce, tomato, onion, carrot

• **Phase 2:** Ask for ½ order of the Open-Faced Roast Beef with the meat only. On the side, order a tossed salad without dressing and Sweet Whole Baby Carrots.

• **Phase 3:** Reduce the beef by 1 ounce, or about 2 tablespoons. Add ½ plain baked potato.

Meatloaf

FAT RELEASERS: beef, tomato, onion, bell pepper, lettuce, carrot

• **Phase 2:** Have ½ order of the Meatloaf with the meat only, plus a tossed salad without dressing and Sweet Whole Baby Carrots.

• **Phase 3:** Reduce the beef by 1 ounce, or about 2 tablespoons, and add ½ cup of Mashed Potatoes.

Oven-Roasted Turkey Breast

FAT RELEASERS: turkey, lettuce, tomato, onion, carrot, green beans

• **Phase 2:** Ask for ½ order of the Oven-Roasted Turkey Breast with the meat only. On the side, order a tossed salad, Sweet Whole Baby Carrots, and Country Green Beans.

• **Phase 3:** Reduce the turkey by 1 ounce, or about 2 tablespoons, and add 1 slice of bread.

Grilled Chicken Tenderloin

FAT RELEASERS: chicken, lettuce, tomato, onion, green beans

• **Phase 2:** Have ½ order of the Grilled Chicken Tenderloin, meat only, plus 2 orders of the tossed salad without dressing and an order of Country Green Beans.

• **Phase 3:** Reduce the chicken by 1 ounce, or about 2 tablespoons, and add 1 slice of bread.

● WARNING! Fat Increaser Ahead

Hunger can undo the best intentions and distract you from your most important job when eating out—ordering a healthy Digest Diet meal. To quiet your stomach, you can nibble on veggies before you leave home or immediately request raw veggies or vegetable or tomato juice as soon as you're seated.

Oven Roasted Turkey Salad

FAT RELEASERS: turkey, egg, lettuce, tomato, onion, cheese
● **Phase 2:** Ask for ½ order of the Oven Roasted Turkey Salad with no croutons or dressing. Add 2 ounces of extra turkey breast.
● **Phase 3:** Reduce the turkey by 1 ounce, or about 2 tablespoons. Add 1 slice of bread.

Grilled Chicken Salad

FAT RELEASERS: chicken, egg, lettuce, tomato, onion, cheese
● **Phase 2:** Eat half of your Grilled Chicken Salad but have all the chicken, and skip the croutons and dressing.
● **Phase 3:** Reduce the chicken by 1 ounce, or about 2 tablespoons, and add 1 slice of bread.

Lemon Pepper Grilled Rainbow Trout

FAT RELEASERS: fish, lemon, pepper, lettuce, tomato, onion, green beans
● **Phase 2:** Order the Lemon Pepper Grilled Rainbow Trout with the fish only. On the side, order a tossed salad without dressing and Country Green Beans.
● **Phase 3:** Reduce the fish by 1 ounce, or about 2 tablespoons, and add ½ plain baked potato.

CULVER'S

- More than 428 restaurants across the country
- (608) 643-7980; www.culvers.com

We had so much fun playing with the Culver's *MyMeal* Nutrition Manager—for every menu item, you can click on the calculator to see what happens nutritionally when you customize your order. Remember to ask for exactly what you want so that you avoid fat increasers such as butter and dressing. Culver's soup menu for Phase 1 is ample (they have more carbs than is ideal for this phase but are much better than other offerings) but varies from restaurant to restaurant.

> **Fun Fat Fact**
>
> Half a cup of split peas has more protein than an ounce of meat, plus one-third of the daily fiber recommendation.

George's Chili

FAT RELEASERS: beans, beef, tomato, bell pepper, chile pepper
- **Phase 1:** Ask for a bowl of George's Chili.
- **Phases 2 and 3:** No change

Stuffed Green Pepper Soup

FAT RELEASERS: bell pepper, beef, tomato, onion
- **Phase 1:** Ask for a bowl of Stuffed Green Pepper soup without rice.
- **Phases 2 and 3:** No change

Split Pea with Ham Soup

FAT RELEASERS: peas, carrot, ham
- **Phase 1:** Order a bowl of Split Pea with Ham Soup.
- **Phases 2 and 3:** No change

Baja Chicken Enchilada Soup

FAT RELEASERS: chicken, tomato, onion, beans, bell pepper, chile pepper
- **Phase 1:** Order a bowl of Baja Chicken Enchilada soup.
- **Phases 2 and 3:** No change

Lumberjack Mixed Vegetable Soup

FAT RELEASERS: tomato, celery, green beans, peas, onion
- **Phase 1:** Order 2 bowls of Lumberjack Mixed Vegetable soup without potatoes.
- **Phases 2 and 3:** No change

Minestrone

FAT RELEASERS: tomato, celery, carrot, green bean, beans, onion, zucchini, spinach
- **Phase 1:** Ask for 3 bowls of Minestrone without potato or macaroni.
- **Phases 2 and 3:** No change

Tomato Florentine Soup

FAT RELEASERS: tomato, zucchini, carrot, celery, spinach
- **Phase 1:** Ask for 1 bowl of Tomato Florentine soup.
- **Phases 2 and 3:** No change

Beef Patty

FAT RELEASERS: beef, lettuce, cucumber, tomato, pea pods, cheese
- **Phase 2:** Order 2 beef patties plus a Garden Fresco Salad with no dressing or croutons.
- **Phase 3:** Eliminate ½ beef patty. Add ½ bun.

Beef Pot Roast Sandwich

FAT RELEASERS: beef, tomato, spinach, lettuce, cucumber, pea pods, cheese
- **Phase 2:** Order the Beef Pot Roast Sandwich with no bun, Tomato Florentine Soup, and a Garden Fresco Salad without dressing or croutons.
- **Phase 3:** Reduce the beef by 1 ounce, or about 2 tablespoons, and add ½ cup of mashed potatoes.

Garden Fresco Salad with Grilled Chicken

FAT RELEASERS: chicken, lettuce, cucumber, tomato, pea pods, cheese, bell pepper, beef

• **Phase 2:** Ask for the Garden Fresco Salad with Grilled Chicken, but skip the croutons and dressing. Add 1 bowl of Stuffed Green Pepper with Beef Soup without rice.

• **Phase 3:** Reduce the chicken by 1 ounce, or about 2 tablespoons, and add 1 dinner roll.

Grilled Chicken Breast

FAT RELEASERS: chicken, vegetables, lettuce, cucumber, tomato, pea pods, cheese

• **Phase 2:** Ask for the Grilled Chicken Breast, 1 cup of Lumberjack Mixed Vegetable Soup, and a Garden Fresco Salad without dressing or croutons.

• **Phase 3:** Reduce the chicken by 1 ounce, or about 2 tablespoons, and add 1 dinner roll.

WARNING! Fat Increaser Ahead

The beef cuts used for sandwiches can range from lean to fatty. According to the National Cattlemen's Beef Association, the leanest cuts of beef are sirloin and round, the traditional roast beef cut.

DEL TACO

● More than 530 restaurants in 17 states
● (800) 852-7204; www.deltaco.com

A classic fast-food taco outlet and the second largest such chain in the US, Del Taco offers a very limited menu, especially for Phase 2. Ask the person taking your order whether you can have a custom-made plate with beef, grilled chicken or steak (plenty of protein spiced up with Digest Diet–friendly seasonings); plus extra lettuce, tomato, and onions (for vitamin C and fiber); and a dollop each of beans and cheese. Salsa always is a good add-on for vitamin C and fat releaser seasoning. Add a small taco-size tortilla for Phase 3. The website offers nutrition info on full meals but not on individual components.

> **Fun Fat Fact**
> Avocados, along with olives and coconuts, are the only fruits that have fat, and all of it is healthy.

● WARNING! Fat Increaser Ahead
Although many brands of corn tortillas can be considered whole grains, they quickly become fat increasers when turned into tortilla chips. Each tortilla can be cut into six or eight chips, and who can stop at so few? Plus the frying process adds oil. To avoid temptation, ask for your meal without chips.

Steak and Egg Burrito

FAT RELEASERS: beef, egg, tomato, cheese, onion
• **Phase 2:** Ask for the Steak and Egg Burrito without the tortilla, plus an order of salsa.
• **Phase 3:** Reduce the beef by 1 ounce, or about 2 tablespoons, and add 1 soft taco-size tortilla.

Classic Taco

FAT RELEASERS: beef, lettuce, cheese, tomato, avocado, onion
• **Phase 2:** Order 2 Classic Tacos, but skip the tortillas. Add 1 dollop of guacamole.
• **Phase 3:** Reduce the beef by 1 ounce, or about 2 tablespoons, and add 1 soft taco-size tortilla.

Taco al Carbon

FAT RELEASERS: beef, tomato, onion, cheese
• **Phase 2:** Ask for 2 Tacos al Carbon with marinated steak without the tortilla, plus 2 tablespoons of cheddar cheese.
• **Phase 3:** Reduce the steak by 1 ounce, or about 2 tablespoons. Add 1 soft taco-size tortilla.

Chicken Asada Taco

FAT RELEASERS: chicken, avocado, tomato, onion
• **Phase 3 only:** Order 2 Chicken Asada Tacos with a dollop of guacamole.

DENNY'S

- Approximately 1,500 locations
- (800) 733-6697; www.dennys.com

Denny's is big on breakfast fare, so we included several breakfast dishes that are suitable for lunch and dinner. Although the chain is traditional American, its menu continuously changes to incorporate international influences and trends. We found a wide range of Digest Diet options, including several items from the Fit Fare menu. You can choose between Denny's nutrition brochure and meal calculator for taking a peek at calories, but you won't be able to customize your meal online.

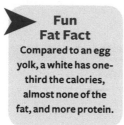

**Fun
Fat Fact**
Compared to an egg yolk, a white has one-third the calories, almost none of the fat, and more protein.

Fit Slam

FAT RELEASERS: eggs, spinach, tomato, fruit, vegetables, broccoli
- **Phase 2:** Ask for the Fit Slam, but skip the bacon and English muffin. On the side, order the Fit Fare Dippable Veggies with no dressing and an order of broccoli.
- **Phase 3:** Decrease to 1 scrambled egg with the Fit Slam vegetables, and add ½ English muffin.

Fit Fare Omelette

FAT RELEASERS: eggs, spinach, tomato, onion, mushroom, fruit, grapes
- **Phase 2:** Ask for the Fit Fare Omelette with no bacon, plus an order of tomato slices and an order of grapes.
- **Phase 3:** Add 1 slice of dinner bread.

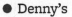

Fit Fare Veggie Skillet

FAT RELEASERS: egg, tomato, spinach, onion, broccoli, mushrooms, bell pepper, green beans, fruit
• **Phase 3 only:** Order the Fit Fare Veggie Skillet with no toast or tortillas. On the side, order green beans and seasonal fruit.

Cranberry Apple Chicken Salad

FAT RELEASERS: chicken, apple, lettuce, fruit
• **Phase 2:** Ask for the Cranberry Apple Chicken Salad without cranberries, pecans, dressing, or bread. Add an order of seasonal fruit.
• **Phase 3:** Add 1 slice of dinner bread.

Avocado Chicken Caesar Salad

FAT RELEASERS: chicken, avocado, cheese, lettuce, grapes
• **Phase 2:** Order the Avocado Chicken Caesar Salad without bacon, dressing, or bread. On the side, have an order of grapes.
• **Phase 3:** Add 1 slice of dinner bread.

Chicken Avocado Sandwich

FAT RELEASERS: chicken, avocado, tomato, onion, lettuce
• **Phase 2:** Ask for the Chicken Avocado Sandwich without bread or sour cream. On the side, order the Garden Salad without dressing.
• **Phase 3:** Add 1 slice of dinner bread.

Tilapia Ranchero

FAT RELEASERS: fish, avocado, tomato, onion, vegetables, broccoli
• **Phase 2:** Order the Tilapia Ranchero without bread or mashed potatoes. On the side, order the Fit Fare Dippable Veggies with no dressing and an order of broccoli.
• **Phase 3:** Reduce the fish by 1 ounce, or about 2 tablespoons, and add ½ cup, about ½ order, of mashed potatoes.

Lemon Pepper Grilled Tilapia

FAT RELEASERS: fish, vegetables, broccoli, grapes
• **Phase 2:** Ask for the Lemon Pepper Grilled Tilapia, fish only, without sauce. On the side, ask for the Fit Fare Dippable Veggies without dressing, an order of broccoli, and an order of grapes.
• **Phase 3:** Reduce the fish by 1 ounce, or about 2 tablespoons. Add ½ cup, about ½ order, of rice pilaf.

DOMINO'S

● 9,000 stores worldwide
● (734) 930-3030; www.dominos.com

Domino's is known for pizza, so you're unlikely to find much else on the menu. Here's where a salad made from pizza toppings becomes your go-to meal. The Domino's website offers a Cal-O-Meter to calculate the calories in your order, but you can't customize based on ingredients.

Salad

FAT RELEASERS: spinach, bell pepper, onion, tomato, cheese, chicken, ham
● **Phase 2:** Make a salad with 1 cup of baby spinach, 1 cup of assorted fresh vegetables, ¼ cup of feta cheese, 2 ounces of grilled chicken breast, and ½ cup of sliced ham.
● **Phase 3:** Reduce the chicken and ham by 1 ounce, or about 2 tablespoons, and add 1 slice of bread.

Mediterranean Veggie Sandwich

FAT RELEASERS: bell pepper, tomato, spinach, onion, cheese.
● **Phase 3 only:** Order the Mediterranean Veggie Sandwich with 1 slice of bread and no provolone or American cheese.

DUNKIN' DONUTS

- 6,772 restaurants in the US and 2,988 international shops in 30 countries
- (781) 737-3000; www.dunkindonuts.com

Most of the Dunkin' Donuts menu is laden with fat increasing carbs and fat, with the exception of a few egg items and an occasional salad. What you can find at Dunkin' Donuts is a wide range of coffee drinks that can be ordered with fat-free milk. The website offers a Printable Nutrition Guide, as well as an on-line Nutrition Catalog of all foods and beverages.

> **Fun Fat Fact**
> The average dough-nut contains at least half its calories from fat and the rest from processed carbs.

Egg and Cheese

FAT RELEASERS: egg, cheese, lettuce, vegetables, milk
- **Phase 2:** Order the egg and cheese without bread, plus a Garden Salad without dressing, and a large (20-ounce) coffee with fat-free milk.
- **Phase 3:** Reduce the egg by 1 ounce, or about 2 tablespoons, and add ½ flatbread.

Egg White Veggie Flatbread

FAT RELEASERS: egg, vegetables, lettuce, milk
- **Phase 3 only:** Ask for the Egg White Veggie Flatbread, a Garden Salad without dressing, and a large (20-ounce) coffee with fat-free milk.

EL POLLO LOCO

- More than 400 restaurants
- (877) 375-4968; www.elpolloloco.com

El Pollo Loco began in Mexico, where the founders grilled fresh chicken marinated in a special recipe of herbs, spices and citrus juices. The chain is all about chicken, a protein-rich menu choice that also delivers vitamin C and fat releaser seasoning. In Phase 2, select your chicken, ditching the fat increasing skin, and pair it with salad vegetables and beans. Top it all off with your choice of four vitamin C–rich salsas. Be very specific when you order, as most items come with fat increaser side dishes such as rice, tortilla chips, and sour cream. If you want to plan your meal ahead, a tool on the company website allows you to see the calories, protein, fiber, vitamin C, and other nutrients in various combinations. For Phase 3, add a tortilla, rice, or mashed potatoes, but watch the portions. The website offers a Nutritional Calculator and a full Nutrition Guide.

> **Fun Fat Fact**
>
> Ordering a tostada salad without the crispy shell immediately saves more than 400 calories.

● **WARNING! Fat Increaser Ahead**

There are different ways to add flavor to grilled meat and poultry, with some increasing fat and others releasing it. Brushing with barbecue sauce is a fat increaser since most sauces are highly sweetened. Pouring sauce over grilled meat before serving adds calories. Dry spice rubs made without sugar add a punch of flavor but almost no calories, while marinating before grilling allows flavors to soak in and calories to drip off.

Chicken Tortilla Soup

FAT RELEASERS: chicken, bell pepper, onion, tomato, cheese, lettuce
- **Phase 2:** Order the large Chicken Tortilla Soup, but skip the tortilla strips. On the side, ask for a large Loco side salad without chips or dressing.
- **Phase 3:** Eliminate the chicken from the soup. Add one 6-inch corn tortilla.

Chicken Tostada Salad

FAT RELEASERS: chicken, lettuce, beans
- **Phase 2:** Ask for an order of the Chicken Tostada Salad without the shell, dressing, sour cream, or rice.
- **Phase 3:** Reduce the chicken by 1 ounce, or about 2 tablespoons, and add one 6-inch corn tortilla.

Grilled Chicken Salad

FAT RELEASERS: chicken, lettuce, corn, tomato, cheese, beans, broccoli, carrot, cauliflower
- **Phase 2:** Ask for an order of the Grilled Chicken Salad without dressing. Ask for an order of pinto beans and fresh vegetables.
- **Phase 3:** Eat half of the beans. Add ½ cup of rice.

Skinless Chicken Breast

FAT RELEASERS: chicken, lettuce, cheese
- **Phase 2:** Remove the skin from an order of Chicken Breast, then add 2 large Loco Side Salads without tortilla strips or dressing.
- **Phase 3:** Reduce the chicken by 1 ounce, or about 2 tablespoons, and add one 6-inch corn tortilla.

Chopped Chicken Breast Meat

FAT RELEASERS: chicken, bell pepper, onion, tomato, beans
- **Phase 2:** Ask for 2 orders of Chopped Chicken Breast Meat. On the side, have 1 small Chicken Tortilla Soup without tortilla strips and ½ order of pinto beans.
- **Phase 3:** Eliminate the beans. Add an order of mashed potatoes.

FIVE GUYS BURGERS AND FRIES

- More than 900 locations nationwide
- (866) 345-GUYS; www.fiveguys.com

> **Fun Fat Fact**
>
> Ounce for ounce, a green pepper tops an orange for vitamin C.

Five Guys has a growing reputation for making great burgers, but there aren't many fat releasers. We grabbed a patty and paired it with as many veggies as we could find.

Burger Patty

FAT RELEASERS: beef, cheese, mushrooms, bell pepper, onion, lettuce, tomato

- **Phase 2:** Order a burger patty, and add a slice of cheese, a cup of lettuce, and ¼ cup each of mushrooms, green peppers, onions, and tomatoes.
- **Phase 3:** Eliminate the cheese, and add ½ bun.

> ● **WARNING!**
> **Fat Increaser Ahead**
> Take time to navigate the topping menu to find the Digest Diet–friendly condiments. Eliminate ketchup, barbecue sauce, relish, and other super-sweet toppings. Say no to grilled veggies; they usually have too much oil. Go for raw vegetables instead, plus mustard, pickles, and salsa if it's available.

FRIENDLY'S

- About 380 locations
- (800) 966-9970; www.friendlys.com

Friendly's offers several classic American dishes and an internationally inspired list of main course salads. In creating the sample meals, we also pulled out the protein portion of a full dinner and then paired it with various combinations of vegetables. We especially like the options on the Build Your Own Burger menu. Friendly's is committed to healthy living and healthy dining, so you'll find nutrition information on the website, as well as suggested healthy meals on the menu.

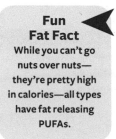

Fun Fat Fact

While you can't go nuts over nuts— they're pretty high in calories—all types have fat releasing PUFAs.

Asian Chicken Salad

FAT RELEASERS: chicken, lettuce, mandarin oranges, almonds, sesame seeds
- **Phase 2:** Order the Asian Chicken Salad without wonton strips or dressing.
- **Phase 3:** Reduce the chicken by 1 ounce, or about 2 tablespoons, and add a slice of bread.

Apple Harvest Chicken Salad

FAT RELEASERS: chicken, apple, walnuts, cheese
- **Phase 2:** Order the Apple Harvest Chicken Salad without dressing.
- **Phase 3:** Reduce the chicken by 1 ounce, or about 2 tablespoons, and add ½ wheat roll.

Chicken Caesar Salad

FAT RELEASERS: chicken, cheese, lettuce, beans
- **Phase 2:** Ask for the Chicken Caesar Salad without dressing or croutons.
- **Phase 3:** Reduce the chicken by 1 ounce, or about 2 tablespoons, and add ½ tomato tortilla.

Savory Chili

FAT RELEASERS: beans, cheese, lettuce
- **Phase 2:** Ask for 1 cup of Savory Chili, ½ order of cheddar cheese, and a side garden salad without dressing.
- **Phase 3:** Eliminate the cheese, and add ½ wheat roll.

Big Beef Burger Patty

FAT RELEASERS: beef, mushrooms, carrot, celery
- **Phase 2:** Order a Big Beef Burger patty, and add an order of sautéed portabella mushrooms and an order of carrot and celery sticks without dressing.
- **Phase 3:** Add ½ wheat roll.

Sirloin Steak Tips

FAT RELEASERS: beef, lettuce, milk
- **Phase 2:** Ask for ½ order of Sirloin Steak Tips with the steak only. Add 2 side orders of the garden salad without dressing and a 1% milk.
- **Phase 3:** Reduce the steak by 1 ounce, or about 2 tablespoons, and add ½ cup of mashed potatoes.

Grilled Chicken Breast

FAT RELEASERS: chicken, bell pepper, carrot, celery, milk
- **Phase 2:** Ask for a grilled chicken breast from the Grilled Chicken BLT, plus green peppers, carrot and celery sticks without dressing, and a 1% milk.
- **Phase 3:** Reduce the chicken by 1 ounce, or about 2 tablespoons, and add ½ tomato tortilla.

Roasted Turkey Dinner

FAT RELEASERS: turkey, bell pepper, broccoli, snap peas, carrot, onion, apple
- **Phase 2:** Order 4 ounces of oven-roasted turkey breast from the Roasted Turkey Dinner (no sides). Add an order of sautéed green peppers, red peppers, broccoli, snap peas, carrot, and red onions. Ask for apple slices on the side.
- **Phase 3:** Reduce the turkey by 1 ounce, or about 2 tablespoons, and add a slice of bread.

GODFATHER'S PIZZA

- More than 600 restaurants in 40-plus states
- (402) 391-1452; www.godfathers.com

As with other pizza chains, Godfather's has mostly pizza on its menu, only one of which is suitable for Phase 3. Luckily, the Godfather's salad bar has an ample selection of Digest Diet–friendly fixings. You also could create a salad from a combination of pizza toppings: artichoke hearts, black beans, garlic, green peppers, jalapeño peppers, lettuce, mushrooms, onions, spinach, tomatoes, cheddar cheese, chicken, ham, Parmesan cheese. Nutritional information on the site includes all types of pizza and salad bar items.

> **Fun Fat Fact**
> According to the 2010 Dietary Guidelines for Americans, ¼ cup of beans is the equivalent in protein to 1 ounce of meat, poultry, or fish.

Salad Bar Salad

FAT RELEASERS: lettuce, vegetables, egg, sunflower seeds, cheese, beans
- **Phase 2:** Have 1 cup of lettuce, 1 cup of vegetables, ¼ cup of egg, ½ ounce (1 tablespoon) of sunflower seeds, 1 ounce (2 tablespoons) of mozzarella cheese, ¼ cup of garbanzo beans, and ¼ cup of kidney beans.
- **Phase 3:** No change

Veggie Pizza (Thin)

FAT RELEASERS: vegetables, spinach, chicken, beans
- **Phase 3 only:** Order 1 medium slice of veggie pie, 1 cup of raw spinach, 1 cup of assorted raw vegetables, ½ cup (2 ounces) of chicken, and ¼ cup of kidney beans.

HARD ROCK CAFÉ

- More than 173 venues
- (407) 445-ROCK; www.hardrock.com

We created our list of Hard Rock meals with a mix of entrée proteins, individual items from combination dishes, and main course salads (that we tinkered with, of course!). Nutrition information is a bit spotty and limited to menus in cities that require posting; New York City is one of them.

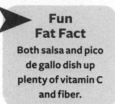

Fun Fat Fact

Both salsa and pico de gallo dish up plenty of vitamin C and fiber.

Honey-Citrus Grilled Chicken Salad

FAT RELEASERS: chicken, orange, lettuce, cheese, bell pepper, pecans

● **Phase 2:** Have ½ order of Honey-Citrus Grilled Chicken Salad without dressing or cranberries.

● **Phase 3:** Add ½ cup of Garlic Herb Smashed Potatoes, while reducing the amount of chicken by 1 ounce, or about 2 tablespoons.

Haystack Chicken Salad

FAT RELEASERS: chicken, lettuce, carrot, corn, tomato, onion, cheese, pecans

● **Phase 2:** Have ½ order of Haystack Chicken Salad, with grilled chicken breast and without dressing and tortilla straws.

● **Phase 3:** Order a 6-inch tortilla, while reducing the amount of chicken by 1 ounce, or about 2 tablespoons.

Cajun Shrimp & Poached Pear Salad

FAT RELEASERS: shrimp, lettuce, cheese, pear, pecans, fruit
● **Phase 2:** Ask for ½ order of Cajun Shrimp & Poached Pear Salad (no bacon or dressing), and ½ order of seasonal fruit.
● **Phase 3:** Add ½ cup of Confetti Rice, while cutting out 2 shrimp.

Grilled Fajita Beef

FAT RELEASERS: beef, tomato, onion, bell pepper, lettuce, vegetables
● **Phase 2:** Ask for ½ order of grilled fajita beef (without the tortilla), 2 tablespoons of pico de gallo, 2 tablespoons of Hard Rock grilled salsa, and 1 side order of house salad (no dressing).
● **Phase 3:** Add one 6-inch tortilla, while reducing the amount of beef by 1 ounce, or about 2 tablespoons.

Classic 6 oz. Burger

FAT RELEASERS: beef, tomato, garlic, basil, vinegar, lettuce, cheese
● **Phase 2:** Have ½ of a burger patty, ½ order of Balsamic Tomato Bruschetta topping (no bread), and 1 side order of Caesar salad (no dressing or croutons).
● **Phase 3:** Add ½ bun.

Grilled Turkey Patty

FAT RELEASERS: turkey, beans, spinach
● **Phase 2:** Ask for ½ of a grilled turkey patty, ½ order of black beans, and 1 large order of raw spinach.
● **Phase 3:** Cut out the beans, and add ½ bun.

Grilled Shrimp

FAT RELEASERS: shrimp, tomato, garlic, basil, balsamic vinegar, lettuce, cheese, avocado
● **Phase 2:** Combine 1 order of grilled shrimp with ½ order of Balsamic Tomato Bruschetta topping (no bread), 1 side order of Caesar salad (no dressing or croutons), and ½ order of avocado slices.
● **Phase 3:** Reduce the amount of shrimp by 1 ounce, or about 2 tablespoons, and add ½ cup of Confetti Rice.

Grilled Salmon

FAT RELEASERS: fish, vegetables, fruit
● **Phase 2:** Ask for ½ order of Grilled Salmon, 1 order of seasonal veggies (no butter or sauce), and ½ order of seasonal fruit.
● **Phase 3:** Reduce the amount of salmon by 1 ounce, or about 2 tablespoons, and add ½ cup of Confetti Rice.

HOOTERS

- More than 430 locations
- www.hooters.com

The Hooters menu

includes lots of bar/pub fare but not many dishes that we could order as is. Our suggested strategy is to pair a protein from the Hooters menu with a salad or veggies from the Build Your Own Burger menu. (There may be an additional charge for this.) Hooters salads, without dressing or croutons, might not be enough food, so we suggest ordering two of them. Phase 3 whole-grain choices are quite limited.

> ◤ **Fun Fat Fact** .
> When you order grilled chicken instead of fried, you get 25% more fat-releasing protein and two-thirds less fat.

Chicken Caesar Salad

FAT RELEASERS: chicken, lettuce, cheese, tomato, cucumber
● **Phase 2:** Have 2 orders of Chicken Caesar Salad without dressing or croutons, and 1 order of Chicken Garden Salad (no dressing).
● **Phase 3:** Add ½ bun, while reducing the amount of chicken by 1 ounce, or about 2 tablespoons.

Grilled Chicken Garden Salad

FAT RELEASERS: chicken, lettuce, cucumber, onion, carrot, bell pepper, mushrooms
● **Phase 2:** Ask for 1 order of Grilled Chicken Garden Salad without dressing or croutons, and 1 cup of assorted Build-a-Burger veggies.
● **Phase 3:** Reduce the amount of chicken by 1 ounce, or about 2 tablespoons, and add ½ bun.

Burger Slider

FAT RELEASERS: beef, cheese, lettuce, cucumber, onion, carrot
- **Phase 2:** Order 1 burger patty, 1 slice of provolone cheese, and ask for 1 order of garden salad (no dressing or croutons).
- **Phase 3:** Eliminate the cheese, and add ½ bun.

Grilled Chicken Breast

FAT RELEASERS: chicken, bell pepper, mushrooms, onion, lettuce, cucumber, carrot
- **Phase 2:** Have the grilled chicken breast from the Grilled Chicken Sandwich plus 1 cup of assorted Build-a-Burger veggies, and 1 order of garden salad (no dressing or croutons).
- **Phase 3:** Reduce the amount of chicken by 1 ounce, or about 2 tablespoons, and add ½ bun.

Grilled Fillet of White Fish

FAT RELEASERS: fish, carrot, celery, lettuce, cucumber, onion
- **Phase 2:** Ask for the grilled fillet of white fish from the Big Fish Sandwich plus 1 order each of carrot sticks and celery sticks without dressing), and 1 order of garden salad (no dressing or croutons).
- **Phase 3:** Add ½ bun, while reducing the amount of fish by 1 ounce, or about 2 tablespoons.

Steamed Shrimp

FAT RELEASERS: shrimp, lettuce, cucumber, onion, carrot
- **Phase 2:** Have 1 order of Steamed Shrimp, no cocktail sauce or butter, and 1 order of garden salad without dressing and croutons.
- **Phase 3:** Add ½ bun, and eliminate 2 shrimp.

Snow Crab Legs

FAT RELEASERS: crab, carrot, celery, lettuce, cucumber, onion
- **Phase 2:** Have ½ order (½ pound) of Snow Crab Legs, 1 order each of carrot sticks and celery sticks without dressing, and 1 order of garden salad (no dressing or croutons).
- **Phase 3:** Reduce the amount of crab by 1 ounce, or about 2 tablespoons, and add ½ bun.

IHOP

- 1,550 IHOP restaurants nationwide
- (866) 444-5144; www.ihop.com

IHOP allows diners to create their own omelette, and that's one of the meals we recommend. Stick with real eggs rather than an egg replacement and pair them with a bit of cheese and an assortment of vegetables. A soup or salad can round out your meal. The IHOP SIMPLE & FIT menu includes lower-calorie options and the SIMPLE & FIT page on the website offers additional tips for slimming down IHOP dishes. The website includes a page with nutritional information on all menu items, including add-ons like cheese and vegetables.

Fun Fat Fact

Skip the egg substitute and go for whole eggs or just whites. They don't have fake ingredients and are filled with fat releasing protein.

WARNING! Fat Increaser Ahead

Big restaurant plates make small portions look downright skimpy. But fill them up and you get way too much food. A 12-inch restaurant plate holds about twice as much as a 9-inch standard dinner plate.

Create Your Own Omelette

FAT RELEASERS: egg, cheese, bell pepper, onion, tomato, spinach, mushrooms, fruit

● **Phase 2:** Have 1 order of Create Your Own Omelette, with 2 eggs, ½ order of Swiss cheese, 1 order each of green peppers and onions, tomatoes, spinach, and mushrooms, and 1 order of seasonal fresh fruit.

● **Phase 3:** Add 1 slice of wheat toast, and eliminate the Swiss cheese.

SIMPLE & FIT Spinach, Mushroom, and Tomato Omelette

FAT RELEASERS: eggs, spinach, mushrooms, tomato, fruit, lettuce, vegetables

● **Phase 2:** Order 1 omelette, and 1 house salad (no dressing).

● **Phase 3:** Ask for the omelette to be made with 1 egg, and add 1 corn tortilla.

SIMPLE & FIT Veggie Omelette

FAT RELEASERS: eggs, vegetables, fruit, tomato, beans

● **Phase 2:** Have 1 order of Minestrone soup, with 1 order of the omelette.

● **Phase 3:** Order 1 slice of wheat toast, while eliminating 1 egg from the omelette.

SIMPLE & FIT Grilled Balsamic-Glazed Chicken

FAT RELEASERS: chicken, vinegar, lettuce, vegetables, fruit

● **Phase 2:** Have 1 order of chicken, 1 order of house salad (no dressing), and 1 order of seasonal fresh fruit.

● **Phase 3:** Reduce the amount of chicken by 1 ounce, or about 2 tablespoons, and add ½ plain baked potato.

SIMPLE & FIT Grilled Tilapia

FAT RELEASERS: fish, lettuce, vegetables, fruit

● **Phase 2:** Ask for 1 order of Grilled Tilapia, 1 order of house salad (no dressing), and 1 order of seasonal fresh fruit.

● **Phase 3:** Reduce the amount of fish by 1 ounce, or about 2 tablespoons, and add ½ plain baked potato.

JACK IN THE BOX

- More than 2,200 quick-serve restaurants in 20 states
- (858) 571-2121; www.jackinthebox.com

Jack in the Box has made a big commitment to nutrition, with extensive nutrition information and suggestions for healthy dining accessible from the website. Also, you can click on and customize menu items to see effects on nutrition. Still, we found vegetables to be in short supply. For Phase 2, your best strategy is to order grilled chicken or a burger patty and pair it with as many vegetables as are available. Jack in the Box, like most fast-food chains, does not yet offer whole grains, so you may need to dip into your Whole Grains To Go Kit (see page 10).

Fun Fat Fact

You get much more than just fat releasing benefits when you eat protein. Protein in a meal helps keep your blood sugar steady, ward off hunger, and conserve muscle.

WARNING! Fat Increaser Ahead

Although the size of fast-food burger patties has stayed about the same since fast food became popular in the 1950s and 1960s, burgers are being made with extra patties and fixings, and portions of fries and beverages are much larger.

Jumbo Jack

FAT RELEASERS: beef, tomato, onion, cheese, lettuce
• **Phase 2:** Ask for 1 Jumbo Jack without the bun, topped with 1 slice of cheese and 1 order of salsa, plus a side salad, no dressing.
• **Phase 3:** Reduce the amount of beef by 1 ounce, or about 2 tablespoons, and add ½ bun.

Sirloin Steak Strips

FAT RELEASERS: beef, chicken, lettuce, tomato, carrot, cucumber
• **Phase 2:** Ask for the sirloin steak strips from the Steak & Egg Burrito, and 1 order Grilled Chicken Salad (no dressing).
• **Phase 3:** Add ½ cup of rice, and reduce the amount of beef by 1 ounce, or about 2 tablespoons.

Chicken Fajita Pita

FAT RELEASERS: chicken, lettuce, onion, cheese, tomato, carrot, cucumber
• **Phase 2:** Order 1 Chicken Fajita, no pita, and 1 Grilled Chicken Salad without dressing.
• **Phase 3:** Reduce the amount of chicken by 1 ounce, or about 2 tablespoons, and add ½ pita.

Southwest Chicken Salad with Grilled Chicken

FAT RELEASERS: chicken, lettuce, beans, onion, tomato, corn, cheese
• **Phase 2:** Have 1 order of Southwest Chicken Salad with Grilled Chicken (with no dressing or corn strips) and 1 order of salsa.
• **Phase 3:** Reduce the amount of chicken by 1 ounce, or about 2 tablespoons, and add ½ pita.

KFC

- More than 5,200 restaurants in the US
- (800) 225-5532; www.kfc.com

There's not a lot for the Digest Diet diner to order at KFC. Still, KFC has been making a push to add and highlight lower-calorie, lower-fat choices like Kentucky Grilled Chicken and a choice of veggie sides. To put together Digest Diet meals, you'll need to remove the skin of your chicken before eating and order more than one side dish to get enough vegetables. KFC tweaks its menu often, so check the KFC Nutrition Guide through the nutrition tab on the website before you go.

Kentucky Grilled Chicken

FAT RELEASERS: chicken, lettuce, cheese, green beans

- **Phase 2:** Order 1 piece of Kentucky Grilled Chicken Breast or 2 pieces of Kentucky Grilled Thigh, removing the skin, and have 1 order of Caesar Side Salad (no dressing or croutons) and 1 order of Green Beans.
- **Phase 3:** Reduce the amount of chicken by 1 ounce, or about 2 tablespoons, and add ½ cup Mashed Potatoes, or a 3-inch Corn on the Cob.

● WARNING! Fat Increaser Ahead

Although they're the smallest part of the chicken, wings can do a lot of diet damage. A single roasted wing—no sauce, no fried coating—has about 100 calories and a fair amount of fat. Breading and frying the wing doubles the calories. Fried skinless wings are not much better.

LEGAL SEA FOODS

- More than 30 locations
- (800) EAT-FISH; www.legalseafoods.com

It's no surprise that the Legal Sea Foods menu is packed with various types of fish. We didn't find as many vegetables, which is why our suggested meals include mainly a salad (we love the sunflower seeds) or broccoli. Very few chain restaurants serve fat releasing quinoa, so we were thrilled to see it here. If you have questions about calorie information, visit the company website and look at the menus in New York or other states, where the information may be required by law.

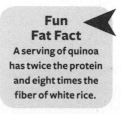

Fun Fat Fact
A serving of quinoa has twice the protein and eight times the fiber of white rice.

Blackened Raw Tuna Sashimi

FAT RELEASERS: fish, lettuce, tomato, carrot, sunflower seeds
- **Phase 2:** Have 1 order of Blackened Raw Tuna Sashimi without the vinaigrette, and ½ order of house salad, no dressing.
- **Phase 3:** Reduce the fish by 1 ounce, or about 2 tablespoons, and add ½ cup of quinoa.

Wood-Burning Grill Rainbow Trout

FAT RELEASERS: fish, bell pepper, lettuce
- **Phase 2:** Ask for 1 order of Wood-Burning Grill Rainbow Trout, no black beans and rice, and 1 order of side salad without dressing.
- **Phase 3:** Reduce the fish by 1 ounce, or about 2 tablespoons, and add ½ cup of black beans and rice.

Haddock

FAT RELEASERS: fish, clams, vegetables, lettuce

• **Phase 2:** Have ½ order of Haddock, along with 1 cup of Lite Clam Chowder, and 1 order of side salad, no dressing.

• **Phase 3:** Reduce the amount of fish by 1 ounce, or about 2 tablespoons, and add ½ cup of quinoa.

Portuguese Fisherman's Stew

FAT RELEASERS: fish, tomato, broccoli

• **Phase 2:** Ask for ½ order of stew and 1 order of broccoli.

• **Phase 3:** Add ½ cup of brown rice, while reducing the amount of fish by 1 ounce, or about 2 tablespoons.

"Fish in Foil"

FAT RELEASERS: fish, vegetables, lettuce, tomato, cucumber, beans, cheese

• **Phase 2:** Have ½ order of fish and ½ order of Chopped Greek Salad, no olives or dressing.

• **Phase 3:** Reduce the amount of fish by 1 ounce, or about 2 tablespoons, and add ½ cup of sweet potatoes.

Rainbow Trout

FAT RELEASERS: fish, lettuce, broccoli

• **Phase 2:** Ask for ½ order of Rainbow Trout, 1 order of side salad without dressing, and 1 order of broccoli.

• **Phase 3:** Add ½ cup of brown rice, while reducing the amount of fish by 1 ounce, or about 2 tablespoons.

Swordfish

FAT RELEASERS: fish, lettuce, broccoli

• **Phase 2:** Have ½ order of Swordfish, 1 order of side salad, no dressing, and 1 order of broccoli.

• **Phase 3:** Reduce the amount of fish by 1 ounce, or about 2 tablespoons, and add ½ cup of quinoa.

Grilled Atlantic Salmon with Tabouli Style Quinoa

FAT RELEASERS: salmon, quinoa, clams, vegetables, lettuce

• **Phase 3 only:** Ask for ½ order of the Grilled Atlantic Salmon with Tabouli Style Quinoa entrée, 1 cup of Lite Clam Chowder, and 1 order of side salad without dressing.

MARIE CALLENDER'S

- 89 Marie Callender's restaurants
- (800) 776-7437; www.mariecallenders.com

The Marie Callender's nutrition calculator is among the best of any restaurant chain—be sure to go online before you dine, pick your meal, and customize it to see the effects on calories and nutrition. Your goal is 425 to 450 calories. In this classically American restaurant, your best options are either a main dish salad or entrée (without fat increasers, of course) or the protein from an entrée paired with a green salad or other veggies. Be as specific as you can about meal components that you don't want on your plate.

> **Fun Fat Fact**
> Chicken breast has slightly fewer calories than chicken thigh meat, along with more protein and less fat.

Rosemary Chicken with Spring Salad

FAT RELEASERS: chicken, lettuce, orange, asparagus, tomato, squash, bell pepper, onion, cauliflower, broccoli, mushrooms

- **Phase 2:** Order the Rosemary Chicken with Spring Salad, but skip the dressing and pecans. Ask for a side order of Roasted Vegetables without cheese.
- **Phase 3:** Reduce the chicken by 1 ounce, or about 2 tablespoons. Add 1 small roll.

Chinese Chicken Salad

FAT RELEASERS: chicken, lettuce, celery, orange, carrot, almond, scallion, asparagus, tomato, squash, bell pepper, cauliflower, broccoli, mushrooms

- **Phase 2:** Ask for the Chinese Chicken Salad without dressing or wontons. Have an order of Roasted Vegetables without cheese.
- **Phase 3:** Reduce the chicken by 1 ounce, or about 2 tablespoons. Add 1 small roll.

"Cabo San Lucas" Chicken Caesar Salad

FAT RELEASERS: chicken, lettuce, tomato, onion, avocado

• **Phase 2:** Order the "Cabo San Lucas" Chicken Caesar Salad without dressing, cheese, or tortilla chips.

• **Phase 3:** Reduce the chicken by 1 ounce, or about 2 tablespoons. Add one 6-inch tortilla.

Gorgonzola, Pecan & Field Greens Salad

FAT RELEASERS: cheese, apple, lettuce, chicken

• **Phase 2:** Ask for ½ order of the Gorgonzola, Pecan & Field Greens Salad with chicken, but skip the dressing, pecans, and cranberries.

• **Phase 3:** Reduce the chicken by 1 ounce, or about 2 tablespoons. Add 1 small roll.

Rosemary Chicken with Potatoes and Broccoli

FAT RELEASERS: chicken, broccoli, fruit

• **Phase 2:** Ask for ½ order of the Rosemary Chicken with Potatoes and Broccoli without potatoes or sauce. Order a side of fresh fruit.

• **Phase 3:** Reduce the chicken by 1 ounce, or about 2 tablespoons, and add ½ cup of mashed potatoes.

Angus Top Sirloin Steak & Asparagus

FAT RELEASERS: beef, asparagus, lettuce, orange

• **Phase 2:** Order the Angus Top Sirloin Steak & Asparagus without onions, mushrooms, butter, or potatoes. Ask for a Spring Salad without dressing or pecans.

• **Phase 3:** Reduce the steak by 1 ounce, or about 2 tablespoons, and add ½ cup of mashed potatoes.

Grilled Chicken Street Tacos

FAT RELEASERS: chicken, cabbage, onion, tomato, lettuce, asparagus, cheese, squash, bell pepper, cauliflower, broccoli, mushrooms

• **Phase 2:** Ask for the Grilled Chicken Street Tacos without dressing or tortillas. On the side, order the Hearts of Romaine with Roasted Vegetables, but skip the dressing.

• **Phase 3:** Reduce the chicken by 1 ounce, or about 2 tablespoons. Add 1 small tortilla.

Freshly Roasted Turkey Dinner

FAT RELEASERS: turkey, vegetables, lettuce, carrot, cabbage, tomato

• **Phase 2:** Order the Freshly Roasted Turkey Dinner with turkey and vegetables only. On the side, have a bowl of Hearty Vegetable Soup and a side Crisp House Salad without dressing or croutons.

• **Phase 3:** Reduce the turkey by 1 ounce, or about 2 tablespoons, and add ½ cup of rice.

Cajun Atlantic Salmon with Broccoli

FAT RELEASERS: salmon, broccoli, shrimp, lettuce, carrot, cabbage, tomato

• **Phase 2:** Ask for ½ order of the Cajun Atlantic Salmon with Broccoli. On the side, have 1 skewer of Cajun Jumbo Shrimp and a Crisp House Salad without dressing or croutons.

• **Phase 3:** Eliminate the shrimp, and add ½ cup of rice.

WARNING! Fat Increaser Ahead

It's human nature to get into patterns of association where one situation triggers another, for example, always ordering pie when eating at a particular restaurant or starting the meal with appetizers when dining out with a particular friend. This can be changed by creating new Digest Diet associations instead. Try walking around the mall instead of having dessert after dinner or start your meal with a salad. The new association will take hold in no time.

Fresh Avocado and Shrimp Stack

FAT RELEASERS: avocado, shrimp, tomato, onion, lettuce, asparagus, cheese, squash, bell pepper, cauliflower, broccoli, mushrooms

• **Phase 2:** Order the Fresh Avocado and Shrimp Stack without dressing or tortilla chips. Ask for an order of Hearts of Romaine with Roasted Vegetables without dressing.

• **Phase 3:** Reduce the shrimp by 2 shrimp. Add 1 small tortilla.

MCDONALD'S

- 33,000 restaurants worldwide
- (800) 244-6227; www.mcdonalds.com

McDonald's leads fast-food chains in its commitment to manage portion sizes and calories and

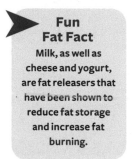

Fun Fat Fact

Milk, as well as cheese and yogurt, are fat releasers that have been shown to reduce fat storage and increase fat burning.

was among the first to offer salads, grilled chicken, fruit, and milk on its menu. Mc-Donald's My Meal Builder on its website allows you to create your own meals and track nutrition. Despite that, there aren't a lot of fat releasing foods on the menu. You may find that once you remove such fat increasers as dressing and buns, your meal is so low in calories that you have to add extra food. McDonald's does not yet have whole grain options yet for Phase 3, so you may want to bring something from the Whole Grains To Go Kit (page 10).

Premium Southwest Salad with Grilled Chicken

FAT RELEASERS: chicken, lettuce, vegetables, cheese, lime, fruit, walnuts

- **Phase 2:** Order the Premium Southwest Salad with Grilled Chicken, and pass on the dressing. On the side, order Snack Size Fruit & Walnuts without yogurt.
- **Phase 3:** Reduce the chicken by 1 ounce, or about 2 tablespoons. Add ½ tortilla.

Quarter Pounder 100% Beef Patty

FAT RELEASERS: beef, chicken, lettuce, tomato, cheese

- **Phase 2:** Order the Quarter Pounder 100% beef patty, plus a Premium Caesar Salad with Grilled Chicken without dressing.
- **Phase 3:** Add ½ bun.

MIMI'S CAFÉ

- close to 60 locations
- (949) 825-7000; www.mimiscafe.com

You'll find a variety of different options on the Mimi's Café menu, including several dishes inspired by various world cuisines. In Phase 2, order your meal without rice or potatoes; you can add a small portion in Phase 3. Ask about entrée salad ingredients and request that fat increasers be left off.

> **Fun Fat Fact**
>
> Foods that are blackened are heavily coated with seasonings—many are fat releasers—and then cooked on the grill or in an iron skillet to char the spice crust.

Asian Chopped Salad

FAT RELEASERS: chicken, cabbage, lettuce, carrot, scallions, bell pepper
- **Phase 2:** Ask for ½ order of the Asian Chopped Salad without wontons or dressing, plus an order of Blackened Chicken.
- **Phase 3:** Reduce the chicken by 1 ounce, or about 2 tablespoons. Add ½ cup of brown rice.

Top Sirloin

FAT RELEASERS: beef, vegetables
- **Phase 2:** Order the Top Sirloin without potatoes, plus an order of Steamed Fresh Vegetables.
- **Phase 3:** Reduce the beef by 1 ounce, or about 2 tablespoons. Add ½ cup of potatoes.

Filet of "Soul"

FAT RELEASERS: fish, vegetables, lettuce, tomato, onion, cheese

• **Phase 2:** Ask for the Filet of "Soul" without rice or potatoes. On the side, order a Petite Wedge without bacon or dressing.

• **Phase 3:** Reduce the fish by 1 ounce, or about 2 tablespoons. Add ½ cup of rice.

Blackened Tilapia

FAT RELEASERS: fish, vegetables

• **Phase 2:** Order the Blackened Tilapia entrée, but skip the rice and potatoes.

• **Phase 3:** Reduce the fish by 1 ounce, or about 2 tablespoons. Add ½ cup of brown rice.

WARNING! Fat Increaser Ahead

Enjoy your 4-ounce glass of wine during or after your meal instead of before. Studies show that people who drink before their meal eat more—alcohol tends to lower inhibitions and makes it harder to put the brakes on. Also, drinkers may not feel as full after eating.

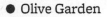

OLIVE GARDEN

- More than 750 local restaurants across the country
- (407) 245-4000; www.olivegarden.com

Olive Garden has popularized Italian food with its extensive menu of traditional dishes and modern interpretations. A favorite chain for feeding the family, Olive Garden dishes out ample portions, along with unlimited salad (yay!) and breadsticks (nope). As at many sit-down restaurants, we recommend eating half portions at Olive Garden, although you may need to make adjustments based on how much you're served. Always ask for your dish to be prepared with less fat and get a full description so that you know whether any ingredients should be left out. You'll find full nutrition info on the restaurant website.

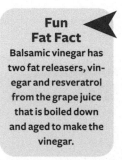

Fun Fat Fact

Balsamic vinegar has two fat releasers, vinegar and resveratrol from the grape juice that is boiled down and aged to make the vinegar.

WARNING! Fat Increaser Ahead

Stay away from breaded, fried fish, where the crusty coating can have more calories than the fish underneath. Steamed oysters and mussels are a tasty alternative with an added bonus—plenty of healthy fat in the form of omega-3 fatty acids.

Steak Toscano

FAT RELEASERS: beef, vegetables, asparagus, vinegar, bell pepper, milk
● **Phase 2:** Order ½ order of the Steak Toscano with grilled vegetables and no potatoes. Have 1 order of asparagus with the balsamic glaze, 1 order of bell peppers, and a cappuccino.
● **Phase 3:** Reduce the amount of beef by 1 ounce, or about 2 tablespoons, and add ½ cup of potatoes.

Venetian Apricot Chicken

FAT RELEASERS: chicken, vegetables, asparagus, vinegar, lettuce
● **Phase 2:** Order ½ order of the Venetian Apricot Chicken with sides of steamed vegetables, asparagus with a balsamic glaze, and the Garden Fresh Salad.
● **Phase 3:** Reduce the amount of chicken by 1 ounce, or about 2 tablespoons, and add ½ cup of pasta.

Grilled Lemon Herb Chicken

FAT RELEASERS: chicken, tomato, spinach, olives, vegetables
● **Phase 2:** Order ½ order of the Grilled Lemon-Herb Chicken with no pasta. Have 1 order of grilled vegetables.
● **Phase 3:** Reduce the amount of chicken by 1 ounce, or about 2 tablespoons, and add ½ cup of potatoes.

Herb-Grilled Salmon

FAT RELEASERS: salmon, broccoli, bell pepper, lettuce, milk
● **Phase 2:** Order ½ of the Herb-Grilled Salmon with broccoli and red peppers and cooked with less oil. Have the Garden Fresh Salad and a cappuccino.
● **Phase 3:** Reduce the amount of salmon by 1 ounce, or about 2 tablespoons, and add ½ cup of rice.

Mussels di Napoli

FAT RELEASERS: fish, tomato, lettuce, milk
● **Phase 2:** Order the Mussels di Napoli. Have the Minestrone Soup, a side order of a green salad, ,and 1 cup of 1% lowfat milk.
● **Phase 3:** Have 1 order of mussels and add 1 small slice of bread.

OUTBACK STEAKHOUSE

- More than 670 restaurants
- (813) 282-1225; www.outback.com

We love the various protein options on the Outback menu, including several cuts and sizes of steaks, chicken, and fish, plus a few entrée salads. Even the petite steaks are big, so you can count on two meals' worth from one order. Order à la carte instead of having a full dinner, and then choose from among several different hot vegetables or pair your protein with a salad.

> **Fun Fat Fact**
> Filet mignon is one of the leanest cuts of beef, and prime rib is among the cuts with the most fat.

Steakhouse Salad

FAT RELEASERS: beef, lettuce, tomato, onion, cheese, vinegar, broccoli
- **Phase 2:** Order ½ of the Steakhouse Salad with no dressing, Aussie Crunch, or pecans. Have 1 order fresh steamed broccoli on the side.
- **Phase 3:** Reduce the amount of steak by 1 ounce, or about 2 tablespoons, and add ½ cup of Garlic Mashed Potatoes.

California Chicken Salad

FAT RELEASERS: chicken, cheese, lettuce, spinach, walnuts, apples
- **Phase 2:** Order the California Chicken Salad with no vinaigrette.
- **Phase 3:** Reduce the amount of chicken by 1 ounce, or about 2 tablespoons, and add 1 small roll.

Victoria's Filet

FAT RELEASERS: beef, vegetables, asparagus

• **Phase 2:** Order ½ Victoria's Filet. Have fresh seasonal mixed veggies and grilled asparagus.

• **Phase 3:** Trim off 1 ounce, or about 2 tablespoons, of beef and add ½ cup of Garlic Mashed Potatoes.

Teriyaki Filet Medallions

FAT RELEASERS: beef, onion, bell pepper, green beans

• **Phase 2:** Order ½ Teriyaki Filet Medallions entrée. Have fresh steamed green beans on the side.

• **Phase 3:** Reduce the amount of beef by 1 ounce, or about 2 tablespoons, and add ½ plain sweet potato.

Grilled Chicken Breast

FAT RELEASERS: chicken, lettuce, vegetables

• **Phase 2:** Eat 4 ounces of grilled chicken breast. Have a house salad with no dressing and fresh seasonal mixed veggies.

• **Phase 3:** Reduce the amount of chicken by 1 ounce, or about 2 table-spoons, and add ½ cup of rice.

Norwegian Salmon

FAT RELEASERS: salmon, vegetables, lettuce, green beans

• **Phase 2:** Order ½ Norwegian Salmon entrée. Have a house salad with no dressing and fresh steamed green beans.

• **Phase 3:** Reduce the amount of fish by 1 ounce, or about 2 tablespoons, and add ½ cup of rice.

Simply Grilled Mahi

FAT RELEASERS: fish, vegetables, broccoli, green beans

• **Phase 2:** Order ½ Simply Grilled Mahi Tuna entrée. Have fresh steamed broccoli and fresh steamed green beans on the side.

• **Phase 3:** Reduce the amount of fish by 1 ounce, or about 2 tablespoons, and add ½ plain baked potato.

Grilled Shrimp on the Barbie

FAT RELEASERS: shrimp, broccoli, green beans, vegetables

• **Phase 2:** Order Grilled Shrimp on the Barbie with no sauce. Have fresh steamed broccoli, fresh steamed green beans, and fresh seasonal mixed veggies.

• **Phase 3:** Leave behind 1 shrimp and add ½ plain sweet potato.

PANDA EXPRESS

- 1,500 restaurants in 42 states
- (800) 877-8988, www.pandaexpress.com

The Panda Express menu has plenty of vegetables in its dishes, and portions are reasonably sized. Unfortunately, not many of the vegetable dishes have enough protein. So your best bets in Phase 2 are any of the Panda Express protein-vegetable main dishes made with sliced or grilled chicken or beef. The word *crispy* is synonymous with breaded and fried, so leave those behind. But it may be possible to swap out the fried ingredients for a more suitable protein such as stir-fried chicken breast strips. The Phase 3 add-on is limited to a small amount of white rice.

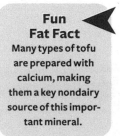

Fun Fat Fact
Many types of tofu are prepared with calcium, making them a key nondairy source of this important mineral.

Panda Express frequently updates its menu, so be sure to check the website ahead of time and ask for descriptions and nutrition information before you order.

WARNING! Fat Increaser Ahead

Porous vegetables like eggplant and mushrooms soak up a lot of fat during cooking, especially if the fat is not hot enough to cook them quickly. If the sauce on your Chinese dish is shiny or has puddles of oil, "wipe off" your veggies by tapping them on extra rice or a small plate to get rid of sauce, fat, and calories.

String Bean Chicken Breast

FAT RELEASERS: chicken, green beans, onion, beef, bell pepper, mushrooms, scallion, sesame seeds, broccoli, cabbage, carrot, zucchini

• **Phase 2:** Order the String Bean Chicken Breast. Also have 1 order of Kobari Beef and a side order of Mixed Veggies.

• **Phase 3:** Reduce the chicken or beef by 1 ounce, or about 2 tablespoons, and add ½ cup of steamed rice.

Mandarin Chicken

FAT RELEASERS: chicken, ginger, tofu, egg, mushrooms, broccoli, cabbage, carrot, green beans, zucchini

• **Phase 2:** Order the Mandarin Chicken. Have the Hot and Sour Soup and a side order of Mixed Veggies.

• **Phase 3:** Reduce the amount of chicken by 1 ounce, or about 2 table-spoons, and add ½ cup of rice.

Black Pepper Chicken

FAT RELEASERS: chicken, celery, onion, black pepper, ginger, beef, broccoli, tofu, egg, mushrooms

• **Phase 2:** Order the Black Pepper Chicken with 1 order of Broccoli Beef and 1 order of the Hot and Sour Soup.

• **Phase 3:** Reduce the amount of chicken or beef to ½ order, and add ½ cup of steamed rice.

Eggplant Tofu

FAT RELEASERS: tofu, bell pepper, eggplant, broccoli, cabbage, carrot, green beans, zucchini

• **Phase 2:** Order the Eggplant Tofu. Have a side order of Mixed Veggies.

• **Phase 3:** Reduce the amount of tofu by 1 ounce, or about 2 tablespoons, and have ½ cup of steamed rice.

PANERA BREAD

- More than 1,500 bakery-cafés in 40 states and Canada
- (314) 984-1000; www.panerabread.com

Like other restaurants with an extensive salad menu, Panera offers several standard salads, along with all the fixings for you to create your own combo. Most salads are well balanced nutritionally and meet Digest Diet guidelines, as long as you order them without dressing or fat increasing extras. If you're in Phase 3, check out Panera's You Pick Two meals, where you can combine two half portions of soup, salad, and/or sandwich. Phase 1 diners have a couple of soups to choose from. Whichever phase you're in, play with the online calculator on the Panera website to customize your meal and see changes in nutrition.

● WARNING!
Fat Increaser Ahead

Remember to order Panera dishes without dressing. Depending on the dressing, the standard 1½ tablespoon portion can add 200 or more calories. Ask for vinegar instead to boost your salad's fat releasing potential.

Low-Fat Vegetarian Garden Vegetable with Pesto Soup

FAT RELEASERS: tomato, zucchini, beans, Swiss chard, cauliflower, bell pepper

- **Phase 1:** Order a large Low-Fat Vegetarian Garden Vegetable with Pesto Soup.
- **Phases 2 and 3:** No change

Low-Fat Vegetarian Black Bean Soup

FAT RELEASERS: beans, onion, bell pepper, garlic, lettuce, tomato, cheese, chile pepper, olives, strawberries, blueberries, pineapple, cantaloupe

● **Phase 1:** Order a large Low-Fat Vegetarian Black Bean Soup.

● **Phase 2:** Order the Low-Fat Vegetarian Black Bean Soup. Have a Greek Salad with no dressing and a Summer Fruit Cup.

● **Phase 3:** Add ½ slice bread.

Strawberry Poppyseed & Chicken Salad

FAT RELEASERS: chicken, lettuce, strawberries, blueberries, pineapple, orange, pecans, milk

● **Phase 2:** Order the Strawberry Poppyseed and Chicken salad with no dressing. Have 1 cup of a cappuccino with fat-free milk.

● **Phase 3:** Reduce the amount of chicken by 1 ounce, or about 2 tablespoons, and add 1 slice of bread.

Fuji Apple Chicken (or Roasted Turkey) Salad

FAT RELEASERS: chicken (or turkey), lettuce, tomato, onion, pecans, cheese, apple

● **Phase 2:** Order the Fuji Apple Chicken Salad or the Roasted Turkey Fuji Apple Salad with no dressing.

● **Phase 3:** Reduce the amount of chicken or turkey by 1 ounce, or about 2 tablespoons, and add 1 slice of bread.

Thai Chopped Chicken Salad

FAT RELEASERS: chicken, lettuce, cashews, edamame, bell pepper, carrot, citrus, nuts, strawberries, blueberries, pineapple, cantaloupe, milk

● **Phase 2:** Order the Thai Chopped Chicken Salad with no dressing or wontons. Have a Summer Fruit Cup and 1 cup of a cappuccino with fat-free milk.

● **Phase 3:** Reduce the amount of chicken by 1 ounce, or about 2 tablespoons, and add 1 slice of bread.

Asian Sesame Chicken Salad

FAT RELEASERS: chicken, lettuce, nuts, sesame seeds, citrus, tomato, zucchini, beans, Swiss chard, cauliflower, bell pepper, basil, strawberries, blueberries, pineapple, cantaloupe

• **Phase 2:** Order the Asian Sesame Chicken Salad with no dressing or wonton strips. Have 1 bowl of the Low-Fat Vegetarian Garden Vegetable with Pesto Soup and a Summer Fruit Cup.

• **Phase 3:** Reduce the amount of chicken by 1 ounce, or about 2 tablespoons, and add 1 slice of bread.

You Pick Two Half Mediterranean Veggie

FAT RELEASERS: lettuce, tomato, onion, cucumber, chile pepper, cheese, beans, bell pepper, garlic, apple

• **Phase 3 only:** Order the You Pick Two Half Mediterranean Veggie on Tomato Basil bread, open-faced, and the You Pick Two Low-Fat Vegetarian Black Bean Soup. Have an apple.

You Pick Two Half Smoked Turkey Breast

FAT RELEASERS: turkey, lettuce, tomato, onion, chicken, avocado, egg, cheese, apple

• **Phase 3 only:** Order the You Pick Two Smoked Turkey Breast on Country, open-faced, and the You Pick Two Half-Chopped Chicken Cobb with Avocado, no dressing or bacon. Have an apple.

You Pick Two Half Roasted Turkey & Avocado BLT

FAT RELEASERS: turkey, avocado, lettuce, tomato, chicken, cheese, apple, milk

• **Phase 3 only:** Order the You Pick Two Half Roasted Turkey & Avocado BLT on Sourdough, open-faced, with no mayo or bacon, and the You Pick Two Half Grilled Chicken Caesar, no dressing or croutons. Have an apple and a caffe latte with fat-free milk.

PAPA JOHN'S

● More than 3,500 restaurants
● (877) 547-PAPA; www.papajohns.com

Papa John's is synonymous with pizza. You'll need to craft your own meal from veggie and other pizza toppings, as there's little else to choose from on the menu.

WARNING!
Fat Increaser Ahead

Beware of "may as well." May as well have an onion ring or three or more. May as well order a specialty beverage and say yes to a refill. May as well let the chef put dressing on the salad. Say "may as well" too many times and your diet efforts will take a hard hit. So remember that every meal offers a new opportunity to eat in a Digest Diet way.

Veggie Combo

FAT RELEASERS: onion, bell pepper, tomato, mushrooms, olives, chicken, cheese

● **Phase 2:** Make your own veggie combo with 2 cups of pizza veggies (onion, bell pepper, tomato, mushrooms, olives), ½ cup of tomato sauce, 1 order of grilled chicken, and ¼ cup of mozzarella cheese.
● **Phase 3:** Add ½ Pizza for One crust.

PEI WEI ASIAN DINER

● (877) 782-6356; www.peiwei.com

A member of the P.F. Chang's family, Pei Wei makes it easy for the Digest Diet follower. You can choose from 12 different sauce-veggie-seasoning combos with different protein options. Several dishes also are available as "stock velveted" rather than stir-fried, a cooking method that reduces fat by up to 30 percent. You can enjoy a "small plate," have a salad, or start your meal with a bowl of soup. Still, you'll need to ask for some items to be left off, such as fried taro (a root vegetable) and rice sticks (a crispy fried noodle). Pay attention to our portion guidelines—most dishes provide two servings.

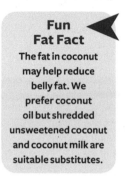

Fun Fat Fact

The fat in coconut may help reduce belly fat. We prefer coconut oil but shredded unsweetened coconut and coconut milk are suitable substitutes.

● **WARNING! Fat Increaser Ahead**

The US interpretation of Chinese food often includes greasy fried meats, oily sauces, and lots of calories. However, some restaurants include steamed options or dishes stir-fried in stock or broth rather than oil, making veggie-centric Chinese fare among the healthiest choices.

Thai Dynamite Beef

FAT RELEASERS: beef, chile pepper, lime, scallions, bell pepper, carrot, soybeans, broccoli, snap peas
• **Phase 2:** Order ½ Thai Dynamite Beef. Have ½ order of the edamame and 1 side order of vegetables.
• **Phase 3:** Reduce the beef by 1 ounce, or about 2 tablespoons, and add ½ cup of brown rice.

Pei Wei Spicy Chicken

FAT RELEASERS: chicken, chile pepper, vinegar, scallions, garlic, snap peas, carrot
• **Phase 2:** Order ½ Pei Wei Spicy Chicken, stock velveted.
• **Phase 3:** Reduce the amount of chicken by 1 ounce, or about 2 tablespoons, and add ½ cup of brown rice.

Sesame Chicken

FAT RELEASERS: chicken, bell pepper, onion, garlic, chile pepper, sesame seeds, broccoli, carrot, snap peas, cabbage
• **Phase 2:** Order half of an order of the Sesame Chicken, stock velveted. Have 1 side order of vegetables and 1 order of the Vietnamese Black Pepper Slaw.
• **Phase 3:** Reduce the amount of chicken by 1 ounce, or about 2 tablespoons, and add ½ cup of brown rice.

Minced Chicken with Cool Lettuce Wraps

FAT RELEASERS: chicken, mushrooms, water chestnuts, scallions, garlic, lettuce
• **Phase 2:** Order ½ order of the Minced Chicken with Cool Lettuce Wraps with no rice sticks.
• **Phase 3:** Reduce the amount of chicken by 1 ounce, or about 2 tablespoons, and add ½ cup of brown rice.

Asian Chopped Chicken Salad

FAT RELEASERS: chicken, lettuce, cabbage, carrot, tomato, sesame seeds
• **Phase 2:** Order ½ order of the Asian Chopped Chicken Salad with no crispy wontons or dressing.
• **Phase 3:** Reduce the amount of chicken by 1 ounce, or about 2 tablespoons, and add ½ cup of brown rice.

Thai Coconut Chicken

FAT RELEASERS: chicken, coconut, ginger, bell pepper, onion, green beans
• **Phase 2:** Order ½ order of the Thai Coconut Chicken.
• **Phase 3:** Reduce the amount of chicken by 1 ounce, or about 2 tablespoons, and add ½ cup of brown rice.

Sesame Vegetables and Tofu

FAT RELEASERS: tofu, bell pepper, onion, garlic, chile pepper, sesame seeds, soybeans

• **Phase 2:** Order ½ order of the Sesame Vegetables and Tofu, stock velveted. Have ½ order of edamame.

• **Phase 3:** Eat ¼ order of edamame and add ½ cup of brown rice.

Ginger Broccoli Shrimp

FAT RELEASERS: shrimp, scallions, ginger, garlic, broccoli, tofu, chile peppers, vinegar, cabbage

• **Phase 2:** Order ½ order of the Ginger Broccoli Shrimp. Have a small cup of the Hot and Sour Soup and 1 order of the Vietnamese Black Pepper Slaw.

• **Phase 3:** Skip the Hot and Sour Soup, and add ½ cup of brown rice.

Spicy Korean Shrimp

FAT RELEASERS: shrimp, chile pepper, garlic, mushrooms, onion, carrot, green beans, sesame seeds, tofu, vinegar, broccoli, snap peas, cabbage

• **Phase 2:** Order ½ order of the Spicy Korean Shrimp. Have a small cup of Hot and Sour Soup, 1 side order of vegetables, and the Vietnamese Black Pepper Slaw.

• **Phase 3:** Skip the soup, and add ½ cup of brown rice.

P.F. CHANG'S CHINA BISTRO

- More than 100 bistros in 32 states
- (866) 732-4264, www.pfchangs.com

P.F. Chang's has an extensive menu loaded with plenty of Phase 2 protein and vegetable options to choose from. But you can't take the menu at face value because it's impossible to know exactly what goes on in the kitchen. If the chef has a heavy hand with oil or cornstarch, your meal quickly could change from fat releaser to fat increaser. So ask that your dish be made with as little oil as possible, or otherwise steamed or sautéed in broth.

> **Fun Fat Fact**
>
> Sesame oil is rich in PUFAs, a type of healthy fat that helps boost metabolism and is burned faster than less healthy saturated fats.

P.F. Chang's serves family style dishes that are meant to feed several people. We've put together a few meals with half orders of various protein-veggie entrées. To turn these into Phase 3 meals, leave behind some of the protein and add ½ cup of brown rice. You also can create your own Phase 2 meal from 4 ounces of lean beef or chicken or 6 ounces of lean fish or seafood plus 2 cups of steamed or stir-fried vegetables, light on the oil.

> **WARNING! Fat Increaser Ahead**
>
> The saturated fat in red meat and full-fat dairy doesn't just increase fat where you can see it on your body. It also pushes its way into cell walls and makes them more susceptible to damage.

Beef with Broccoli

FAT RELEASERS: beef, broccoli, garlic, scallions, ginger
- **Phase 2:** Order ½ order of the Beef with Broccoli.
- **Phase 3:** Reduce the amount of beef by 1 ounce, or about 2 tablespoons, and add 1 steamed pork dumpling with no sauce.

Pepper Steak

FAT RELEASERS: beef, onion, bell pepper, garlic, black pepper
- **Phase 2:** Order ½ order of the Pepper Steak.
- **Phase 3:** Reduce the amount of beef by 1 ounce, or about 2 tablespoons, and add ½ cup of brown rice.

Orange Peel Beef

FAT RELEASERS: beef, orange
- **Phase 2:** Order ½ order of Orange Peel Beef.
- **Phase 3:** Reduce the amount of beef by 1 ounce, or about 2 tablespoons, and add ½ cup of brown rice.

Chengdu Spiced Lamb

FAT RELEASERS: lamb, tomato, onion, egg, carrot, scallions
- **Phase 2:** Order ½ order of the Chengdu Spiced Lamb and 1 order of Egg Drop Soup.
- **Phase 3:** Reduce the amount of lamb by 1 ounce, or about 2 tablespoons, and add ½ cup of brown rice.

Ginger Chicken with Broccoli

FAT RELEASERS: chicken, broccoli, scallions, ginger
- **Phase 2:** Have ½ order of the Ginger Chicken with Broccoli.
- **Phase 3:** Reduce the amount of chicken by 1 ounce, or about 2 tablespoons, and add ½ cup of brown rice.

Asian Grilled Norwegian Salmon

FAT RELEASERS: salmon, asparagus, tofu, vegetables
- **Phase 2:** Order the Asian Grilled Norwegian Salmon with no rice. Have ½ order of Buddha's Feast (steamed with no rice).
- **Phase 3:** Reduce the amount of salmon by 1 ounce, or about 2 tablespoons, and add ½ cup of brown rice.

Norwegian Salmon Steamed with Ginger

FAT RELEASERS: salmon, mushrooms, bok choy, tomato, asparagus, tofu, vegetables
- **Phase 2:** have ½ order of the Norwegian Salmon Steamed with Ginger and one order of Buddha's Feast (steamed with no rice).
- **Phase 3:** Reduce the amount of salmon by 1 ounce, or about 2 tablespoons, and add ½ cup of brown rice.

Shrimp with Lobster Sauce

FAT RELEASERS: shrimp, garlic, black beans, mushrooms, scallions, egg, tofu, vegetables, chicken, vinegar

● **Phase 2:** Have ½ order of the Shrimp with Lobster Sauce. Have 1 order of Buddha's Feast (steamed with no rice) and 1 order of the Hot and Sour Soup.

● **Phase 3:** Eliminate the soup, and add ½ cup of brown rice.

Sichuan Shrimp

FAT RELEASERS: shrimp, chile pepper, garlic, egg, carrot, scallions, snap peas

● **Phase 2:** Have ½ order of the Sichuan Shrimp. Have 1 order of Egg Drop Soup and 1 order of Garlic Snap Peas.

● **Phase 3:** Reduce the amount of shrimp by 2 to 3 shrimp, and add 1 steamed pork dumpling.

PIZZA HUT

- More than 6,000 restaurants
- (800) 948-8488; www.pizzahut.com

You certainly can eat at Pizza Hut during Phase 2, but you'll have to create your meal from a combination of pizza topping vegetables, plus chicken or ham, and sauce if you like. A slice of the smallest size Pizza Hut pizza, plus extra veggies and protein, is suitable for Phase 3.

> **Fun Fat Fact**
> Top your meal with a generous amount of red pepper flakes. Spicy condiments, including chile peppers, hot sauce, and salsa cause your body to burn hotter.

Ham & Pineapple Pizza

FAT RELEASERS: ham, pineapple, vegetables, cheese
- **Phase 3 only:** Order 1 medium slice of the Ham & Pineapple Pizza, Thin 'N Crispy. Have 2 cups of assorted veggies.

Ham, Pineapple & Diced Red Tomato Pizza

FAT RELEASERS: ham, pineapple, tomato, vegetables, cheese
- **Phase 3 only:** Order 1 medium slice of the Ham, Pineapple & Diced Red Tomato Pizza, Fit 'N Delicious. Have 1 order of extra ham and 2 cups of assorted veggies.

Chicken, Red Onion & Green Pepper Pizza

FAT RELEASERS: chicken, onion, bell pepper, vegetables, cheese
- **Phase 3 only:** Order 1 medium slice of the Chicken, Red Onion & Green Pepper Pizza, Fit 'N Delicious topped with 1 order of extra chicken and 2 cups of assorted veggies.

Veggie Lover's Pizza

FAT RELEASERS: vegetables, cheese
- **Phase 3 only:** Order 1 medium slice of the Veggie Lover's Pizza, Thin 'N Crispy. Have 2 cups of assorted veggies.

QDOBA MEXICAN GRILL

● More than 200 restaurants
● (720) 898-2300; www.qdoba.com

Qdoba allows you to mix and match to create your own customized meal, so feel free to choose from grilled steak and chicken for protein, two types of fiber-rich beans, grilled vegetables for fiber and vitamin C, lettuce, and salsas packed with vitamin C and seasonings. For healthy fats, add a dollop of guacamole. You can visit the Qdoba website to check out the calories and fat in the various combinations you create.

> **Fun Fat Fact**
> Compared to sour cream, guacamole has less than half the amount of unhealthy saturated fat, along with more fiber and vitamin C.

WARNING! Fat Increaser Ahead

It's more important to swap unhealthy fats for healthy fats in moderation than to cut out as much fat as possible. MUFA-rich guacamole is a better choice than sour cream and MUFA-rich olives are a smarter pick than fried tortilla strips. But all fats are high in calories, so portion management is critical.

Taco Salad

FAT RELEASERS: lettuce, beef, tomato, onion, bell pepper, zucchini, squash, avocado
• **Phase 2:** Order a Taco Salad with lettuce, seasoned ground beef, pico de gallo, fajita vegetables, and guacamole.
• **Phase 3:** Reduce the amount of beef by 1 ounce, or about 2 tablespoons, and add ½ whole wheat tortilla.

Mexican Platter

FAT RELEASERS: beans, bell pepper, zucchini, squash, beef, chile pepper, corn
• **Phase 2:** Create your own platter with black beans, grilled vegetables, grilled steak, and roasted chile-corn salsa.
• **Phase 3:** Replace the beans with ½ of a whole wheat tortilla.

Mexican Gumbo

FAT RELEASERS: tomato, beans, chicken, onion
• **Phase 2:** Order the Mexican Gumbo with Tortilla Soup with no rice or tortilla strips, plus pinto beans, grilled chicken, and salsa roja.
• **Phase 3:** Replace ½ order of beans with ½ cup of cilantro-lime rice.

WARNING! Fat Increaser Ahead

Refried beans are not fried twice, just once or not at all. But depending on the restaurant, they can be high in calories and fat. They're often prepared with lard and sometimes with cheese on top or melted in. Some restaurants offer both traditional refried beans and a different type of bean prepared without fat.

Mango Salad

FAT RELEASERS: lettuce, chicken, mango, bell pepper, zucchini, squash, avocado, beans, corn
• **Phase 2:** Order a Mango Salad with lettuce, grilled chicken, mango salsa, grilled vegetables, guacamole, and black bean and corn salsa.
• **Phase 3:** Replace the black bean and corn salsa with ½ cup of cilantro-lime rice.

QUIZNOS

- More than 4,000 locations
- (720) 359-3300; www.quiznos.com

Quiznos is a pretty standard sandwich shop with the usual fixings, plus a rotating menu of seasonal and new ingredients. What we especially like is that Quiznos encourages patrons to pick their own ingredients and choose from small and large portions, so enjoy customizing your salad or breadless sandwich. Quiznos offers wheat bread, a perfect addition for Phase 3. Visit the Quiznos website to look at nutrition information and learn about new menu items.

> **Fun Fat Fact**
>
> The sandwich shop menu has more types of fat releasing lean proteins—beef, chicken breast, turkey breast, and ham—than most other types of restaurants.

Honey Mustard Chicken Salad

FAT RELEASERS: chicken, lettuce, tomato, cheese, beans, beef
- **Phase 2:** Order 1 large Honey Mustard Chicken Salad with no dressing or bacon. Have 1 small bowl of Chili.
- **Phase 3:** Reduce the amount of chicken by 1 ounce, or about 2 tablespoons, and add ½ small Artisan Wheat bread.

Cobb Salad

FAT RELEASERS: lettuce, chicken, egg, tomato, cheese
- **Phase 2:** Order 1 large Cobb Salad with no dressing or bacon, plus 4 ounces of chicken breast.
- **Phase 3:** Reduce the amount of chicken by 1 ounce, or about 2 tablespoons, and add ½ small Artisan wheat bread.

Peppercorn Caesar Salad with Chicken

FAT RELEASERS: lettuce, chicken, tomato, cheese

• **Phase 2:** Order 1 large Peppercorn Caesar Salad with Chicken, no dressing, plus 4 ounces of chicken breast.

• **Phase 3:** Reduce the amount of chicken by 1 ounce, or about 2 tablespoons, and add ½ small Artisan Wheat bread.

Mediterranean Chicken Salad

FAT RELEASERS: lettuce, chicken, tomato, cucumber, chile pepper, beans, cheese, olives

• **Phase 2:** Order 1 large and 1 small Mediterranean Chicken Salad with no dressing.

• **Phase 3:** Reduce the amount of chicken by 1 ounce, or about 2 tablespoons, and add ½ small Artisan Wheat bread.

Roast Beef

FAT RELEASERS: beef, cheese, lettuce, tomato, onion, bell pepper

• **Phase 2:** have 1 large order of Roast Beef. Have 1 small slice of mozzarella cheese, and 1 large order each of lettuce, tomatoes, onions, and peppers.

• **Phase 3:** Reduce the amount of beef by 1 ounce, or about 2 tablespoons, and add ½ small Artisan Wheat bread.

Turkey Breast

FAT RELEASERS: turkey, cheese, avocado, lettuce, tomato, onion, bell pepper

• **Phase 2:** Have 1 large order of the Turkey Breast. Have 1 small slice of Swiss cheese, 1 order of guacamole, and 1 large order each of lettuce, tomatoes, onions, and peppers.

• **Phase 3:** Reduce the amount of turkey by 1 ounce, or about 2 tablespoons, and add ½ small Artisan Wheat bread.

Chicken Breast

FAT RELEASERS: chicken, cheese, lettuce, tomato, onion, bell pepper

• **Phase 2:** Order 4 ounces of Chicken Breast. Have 1 small slice of cheddar cheese, and 1 large order each of lettuce, tomatoes, onions, and peppers.

• **Phase 3:** Reduce the amount of chicken by 1 ounce, or about 2 tablespoons, and add ½ small Artisan Wheat bread.

Lobster & Seafood Salad

FAT RELEASERS: seafood, lettuce, tomato, avocado, onion, bell pepper

• **Phase 2:** Order 1 large Lobster & Seafood Salad with no dressing. Have 1 order of guacamole and 1 large order each of lettuce, tomatoes, onions, and peppers.

• **Phase 3:** Reduce the amount of seafood by 1 ounce, or about 2 tablespoons, and add ½ small Artisan Wheat bread.

RED LOBSTER

- More than 680 locations
- (800) Lobster; www.redlobster.com

Red Lobster reliably dishes up a variety of different types of fish and seafood, plus steak for non-fish eaters. Here, you can order a full dinner, choosing a salad and a vegetable as your side dishes. Give blackened fish a try—the crusty spices do double-duty as fat releasers. The Red Lobster menu changes frequently, so be sure to read the menu and order only what you want. You can find several pages of nutrition information on the Red Lobster website.

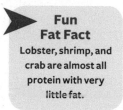

Fun Fat Fact

Lobster, shrimp, and crab are almost all protein with very little fat.

⚫ WARNING! Fat Increaser Ahead

How often do you leave a restaurant feeling overly full? Do you find that your restaurant meals are over in an hour? Eating quickly can cause you to blow through your body's fullness signals without stopping when you've had enough. You can slow down the pace of your meal and be better able to respond to fullness cues by picking foods that require a bit of work to eat, for example, cracking crabs or pulling the meat out of lobster claws.

Wood-Grilled Peppercorn Sirloin and Shrimp

FAT RELEASERS: beef, shrimp, lettuce, vegetables, asparagus
• **Phase 2:** Have ½ order of the Wood-Grilled Peppercorn Sirloin and Shrimp with no butter or mashed potatoes. Have a Garden Salad with no dressing and 1 order of fresh asparagus.
• **Phase 3:** Reduce the amount of steak by 1 ounce, or about 2 tablespoons, and add ½ plain baked potato.

Center-Cut NY Strip Steak

FAT RELEASERS: beef, clams, tomato, asparagus
• **Phase 2:** Have ½ order of the Center-Cut NY Strip Steak. Have 1 bowl of the Manhattan Clam Chowder and 1 order of fresh asparagus.
• **Phase 3:** Reduce the amount of steak by 1 ounce, or about 2 tablespoons, and add ½ plain baked potato.

Grilled Fresh Salmon

FAT RELEASERS: salmon, lettuce, vegetables, broccoli
• **Phase 2:** Order the Grilled Fresh Salmon. Have a Garden Salad with no dressing and 1 order of fresh broccoli.
• **Phase 3:** Reduce the amount of salmon by 1 ounce, or about 2 tablespoons, and add ½ cup of wild rice pilaf.

Oven-Broiled Fish

FAT RELEASERS: fish, lettuce, vegetables
• **Phase 2:** Order the Oven-Broiled Fish. Have a Garden Salad with no dressing.
• **Phase 3:** Reduce the amount of fish by 1 ounce, or about 2 tablespoons, and add ½ plain baked potato.

Blackened Tilapia

FAT RELEASERS: fish, broccoli, asparagus
• **Phase 2:** Have the Blackened Tilapia with 1 order of fresh broccoli and 1 order of fresh asparagus.
• **Phase 3:** Reduce the amount of fish by 1 ounce, or about 2 tablespoons, and add ½ cup of wild rice pilaf.

Garlic-Grilled Shrimp Skewer

FAT RELEASERS: shrimp, garlic, clams, tomato, lettuce, vegetables
• **Phase 2:** have 2 orders of the Garlic-Grilled Shrimp Skewer. Have 1 bowl of Manhattan Clam Chowder and a Garden Salad with no dressing.
• **Phase 3:** Reduce the amount of shrimp by ½ skewer, and add ½ cup of rice.

Snow Crab Legs

FAT RELEASERS: crab, clams, tomato, lettuce, vegetables, broccoli
● **Phase 2:** Order the Snow Crab Legs. Have 1 bowl of Manhattan Clam Chowder, a Garden Salad with no dressing, and 1 order of fresh broccoli.
● **Phase 3:** Reduce the amount of crab by 1 ounce, or about 2 tablespoons, and add ½ plain baked potato.

Wood-Grilled Lobster, Shrimp, and Scallops

FAT RELEASERS: seafood, lettuce, vegetables, broccoli
● **Phase 2:** have ½ order of the Grilled Lobster, Shrimp, and Scallops with no butter or wild rice. Have a Garden Salad with no dressing and 1 order of fresh broccoli.
● **Phase 3:** Reduce the amount of shellfish by 1 ounce, or about 2 tablespoons, and add ½ cup of wild rice pilaf.

Steamed Live Main Lobster

FAT RELEASERS: lobster, lettuce, vegetables, asparagus
● **Phase 2:** Order the Steamed Live Maine Lobster. Have a Garden Salad with no dressing and 1 order of fresh asparagus.
● **Phase 3:** Reduce the amount of lobster by 1 ounce, or about 2 tablespoons, and add ½ cup of wild rice pilaf.

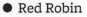

RED ROBIN

● More than 400 restaurants nationwide
● (303) 846-6000; www.redrobin.com

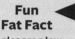

Red Robin is known for its burgers—not just beef but also chicken and turkey. Main course salads fill out the menu, meaning that you'll find plenty of dishes to choose from. Before dining at Red Robin, visit its website, access the nutrition tool, and play around with different food combinations to see the nutrition changes. Choose the whole-grain bun in Phase 3; eat one quarter of a bun, as the buns are large.

**Fun
Fat Fact**

Apples are a low-glycemic food that has only a small effect on blood glucose and insulin levels. In addition to fiber, apples are rich in antioxidants.

Simply Grilled Chicken Salad

FAT RELEASERS: chicken, lettuce, cucumber, tomato, cheese, vegetables
● **Phase 2:** Order the Simply Grilled Chicken Salad with no croutons, dressing, or bread. Have 1 order of the Chicken Tortilla Soup with no tortillas.
● **Phase 3:** Skip the soup, and add 1 small piece of garlic focaccia bread.

Apple Harvest Chicken Salad

FAT RELEASERS: chicken, lettuce, apple, cheese, beans
● **Phase 2:** Order the Apple Harvest Chicken Salad with no dressing, walnuts, or bread. Have 1 order of Southwest Black Beans.
● **Phase 3:** Reduce the amount of chicken by 1 ounce, or about 2 tablespoons, and add ¼ whole-grain bun.

● The Digest Diet Dining Out Guide

Southwest Grilled Chicken Salad

FAT RELEASERS: chicken, lettuce, vegetables, beans, corn, avocado, lime, fruit

• **Phase 2:** Order the Southwest Grilled Chicken Salad with no dressing, tortilla strips, cheese, or fried jalapeño rings. Have the Freckled Fruit Salad.

• **Phase 3:** Reduce the amount of chicken by 1 ounce, or about 2 tablespoons, and add ½ cup of Southwestern Rice.

Lettuce-Wrap Your Burger

FAT RELEASERS: beef, lettuce, tomato, onion, vegetables

• **Phase 2:** Order the Lettuce-Wrap Your Burger with no cheese and a House Salad with no dressing.

• **Phase 3:** Add ¼ of a whole grain bun.

California Chicken Sandwich

FAT RELEASERS: chicken, avocado, lettuce, tomato, onion, vegetables, cheese, fruit

• **Phase 2:** Order the California Chicken Sandwich with no bun, bacon, or mayonnaise. Have 1 order of Chicken Tortilla Soup with no tortillas and 1 order of the Freckled Fruit Salad.

• **Phase 3:** Reduce the amount of chicken by 1 ounce, or about 2 tablespoons, and add ¼ whole-grain bun.

Grilled Turkey Burger

FAT RELEASERS: turkey, lettuce, tomato, onion, vegetables, broccoli

• **Phase 2:** Order the Grilled Turkey Burger with no bun or mayo. Have a Side Salad with no dressing and 1 order of steamed broccoli.

• **Phase 3:** Add ¼ whole-grain bun.

Ensenada Chicken Platter

FAT RELEASERS: chicken, lettuce, cheese, tomato, onion, lime, broccoli

• **Phase 2:** Order the Ensenada Chicken Platter with no tortilla strips or dressing. Have 1 order of steamed broccoli.

• **Phase 3:** Reduce the amount of chicken by 1 ounce, or about 2 tablespoons, and add ½ cup of Southwestern Rice.

Hummus Plate

FAT RELEASERS: beans, carrot, cucumber, jicama, zucchini, vegetables, cheese, fruit

• **Phase 2:** Have ½ order of the Garden Fresh Hummus Plate with no olive oil or bread. Have 1 order of the Roasted Vegetable Soup with no garlic bread and the Freckled Fruit Salad.

• **Phase 3:** Reduce the amount of hummus by 2 tablespoons and add 1 small piece of garlic focaccia bread.

ROMANO'S MACARONI GRILL

- 222 locations in the U.S. and internationally
- (972) 674-4300; www.romanosmacaronigrill.com

At Romano's Macaroni Grill, choose entrées à la carte and add the side dishes that you want, or make your own dish from the Create Your Own Pasta menu (no pasta except in Phase 3, of course). The nutrition information page on the website includes calories and nutrients for all dishes, including each item on the pasta menu.

> **Fun Fat Fact**
> Every ½ cup of cooked pasta is the grain equivalent to a slice of bread. Whole-grain pasta has much more fiber than traditional pasta does.

⬤ WARNING! Fat Increaser Ahead

People tend to keep putting more food on their plate when food is in easy reach in family-style bowls and platters. A smarter approach is to dish out the appropriate portion and avoid going back for seconds or picking at what's left in the bowl.

Sliced Turkey Breast

FAT RELEASERS: turkey, tomato, lettuce

• **Phase 2:** Eat 4 ounces of Sliced Turkey Breast with 1 order of the Pomodorina Soup and 1 order of the Caesar Salad with no dressing.

• **Phase 3:** Reduce the turkey by 1 ounce, or about 2 tablespoons, and add 1 small slice of bread.

Carmela's Chicken

FAT RELEASERS: chicken, lettuce, vegetables

• **Phase 2:** Have ½ order of Carmela's Chicken. Have a Fresh Greens Salad with no dressing and 2 cups of assorted vegetables.

• **Phase 3:** Reduce the amount of chicken by 1 ounce, or about 2 tablespoons, and add ½ cup of whole-wheat pasta.

Grilled Chicken Spiedini (Skewer)

FAT RELEASERS: chicken, vegetables

• **Phase 2:** Order the Grilled Chicken Spiedini (Skewer).

• **Phase 3:** Reduce the amount of chicken by 1 ounce, or about 2 tablespoons, and add ½ cup of whole-wheat pasta.

Create Your Own Pasta

FAT RELEASERS: vegetables, beans, chicken

• **Phase 2:** From the Create Your Own Pasta menu, order 2 cups of assorted vegetables, ½ cup of cannellini beans and 4 ounces of roasted chicken.

• **Phase 3:** Reduce the amount of chicken by 1 ounce, or about 2 tablespoons, and add ½ cup of whole-wheat pasta.

Grilled Shrimp Spiedini (Skewer)

FAT RELEASERS: shrimp, vegetables

• **Phase 2:** Order the Grilled Shrimp Spiedini (Skewer).

• **Phase 3:** Reduce the amount of shrimp by 2 shrimp, and add ½ cup of whole-wheat pasta.

Goat Cheese Peppadew Peppers

FAT RELEASERS: chile pepper, cheese, lettuce, mushrooms

• **Phase 2:** Have ½ order of the Goat Cheese Peppadew Peppers. Have a side order of the Fresh Greens Salad with no dressing and 1 order of the Roasted Mushroom Soup.

• **Phase 3:** Skip the mushroom soup and add 1 small slice of bread.

RUBY TUESDAY

- About 750 locations
- (865) 380-7603; www.rubytuesday.com

What we like about Ruby Tuesday is that every entrée comes with a trip to the Create Your Own Garden Bar, an extensive salad bar. We encourage you to visit the bar and put together an entrée or side salad, depending on the rest of your order. Feel free to swap out any of the vegetables in our sample meals for a salad of your own creation.

> **Fun Fat Fact**
> Sniff or visualize eating a favorite food, and you'll feel less hungry.

● WARNING! Fat Increaser Ahead

Whether it's the bowl of chips on the table, the frosty glasses of margaritas, or the crispy fried appetizers, aspects of the restaurant environment are engineered to entice diners into ordering more food. Take control of your environment by asking to have the chips taken away, requesting a tall glass of ice water as soon as you sit down, and skipping the appetizer section of the menu altogether.

Petite Grilled Chicken Salad

FAT RELEASERS: chicken, lettuce, peas, tomato, cucumber, carrot, mushrooms, bell pepper

• **Phase 2:** Order the Petite Grilled Chicken Salad with no bacon, croutons, or dressing. Have 2 Asian Chicken Lettuce Wraps as well.

• **Phase 3:** Order just 1 lettuce wrap, and add ½ plain baked potato.

Chicken Fresco

FAT RELEASERS: chicken, tomato, vinegar, broccoli, green beans

• **Phase 2:** Order the Chicken Fresco with no lemon butter. Have 1 order of Fresh Steamed Broccoli and 1 order of Fresh Grilled Green Beans.

• **Phase 3:** Reduce the amount of chicken by 1 ounce, or about 2 tablespoons, and add ½ cup of brown-rice pilaf.

Turkey Minis

FAT RELEASERS: turkey, lettuce, tomato, green beans, squash

• **Phase 2:** Order 3 Turkey Minis with no mayo or bun. Have 1 order of Fresh Grilled Green Beans and 1 order of Roasted Spaghetti Squash.

• **Phase 3:** Order 2 Turkey Minis, no mayo, and 1 mini bun.

Creole Catch

FAT RELEASERS: fish, zucchini, squash, green beans

• **Phase 2:** Order the Creole Catch with 1 order of Fresh Grilled Green Beans.

• **Phase 3:** Decrease the fish by 1 ounce, or about 2 tablespoons, and add ½ plain baked potato.

Grilled Salmon

FAT RELEASERS: salmon, zucchini, squash, tomato, olive oil, vinegar

• **Phase 2:** Order the Grilled Salmon with 1 order of sliced tomatoes.

• **Phase 3:** Reduce the amount of salmon by 1 ounce, or about 2 tablespoons, and add ½ plain baked potato.

RYAN'S

- More than 300 restaurants
- (864) 879-1000; www.ryans.com

Ryan's, and its sister restaurants Old Country Buf-

fet, HomeTown Buffet, Fire Mountain, and Granny's Buffet, serve food buffet-style, so you are completely in charge of what and how much goes on your plate. We stuck mainly with green salads to be sure that we didn't add too much extra fat to the meals. You can enjoy any salads and veggies that don't look like they're swimming in oil or mayo. Ryan's nutrition information is based on a serving spoon—we used that same measure in planning your meals.

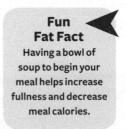

Fun Fat Fact

Having a bowl of soup to begin your meal helps increase fullness and decrease meal calories.

⬤ WARNING! Fat Increaser Ahead

With big plates and plenty of calorie-laden choices, buffets can be a Digest Diet nightmare. Check out the entire buffet line before making your selections, and limit your choices to dishes that are not dripping with dressing or sauce. Use your best portion management skills to put the right amount of food on your plate.

Minestrone Soup

FAT RELEASERS: beans, vegetables, lettuce, egg, cheese, turkey, grapes
- **Phase 1:** Have 4 ladles (2 cups) of Minestrone Soup.
- **Phase 2:** Dish out 2 ladles (1 cup) of Minestrone Soup. Create a chef salad with 2 cups of romaine lettuce, 4 spoons of assorted raw veggies, 2 spoons of diced eggs, 2 spoons of cottage cheese, 3 ounces of turkey breast, and 1 spoon of grapes.
- **Phase 3:** Skip the cottage cheese, and add 1 slice wheat bread.

Chili Bean Soup

FAT RELEASERS: beans, vegetables, lettuce, cheese, broccoli, chicken, tomato, onion, avocado
- **Phase 1:** Dish up 4 ladles (2 cups) of Chili Bean Soup.
- **Phase 2:** Serve yourself 2 ladles (1 cup) of the Chili Bean Soup. Make a taco salad with 2 cups of Spring Mix, 1 spoon of shredded cheese, 1 spoon of broccoli florets, 2 spoons of chicken taco meat, 1 spoon of diced taco bar veggies, 2 spoons of guacamole, and 1 ladle of pico de gallo.
- **Phase 3:** Skip the shredded cheese, and add ½ cup rice.

Carved Roast Beef

FAT RELEASERS: beef, lettuce, vegetables
- **Phase 2:** Have 4 ounces of the Carved Roast Beef, 2 cups of romaine lettuce and 4 spoons of assorted raw veggies.
- **Phase 3:** Reduce the amount of beef by 1 ounce, or about 2 tablespoons, and add 1 slice wheat bread.

Carved Sirloin Steak

FAT RELEASERS: beef, beans, lettuce, vegetables
- **Phase 2:** Serve yourself 4 ounces of the Carved Sirloin Steak. Have 2 ladles (1 cup) of the Chili Bean Soup, 2 cups of romaine lettuce, and 4 spoons of assorted raw veggies.
- **Phase 3:** Reduce the amount of steak by 1 ounce, or about 2 tablespoons, and add ½ cup Mexican Rice.

Oriental Chicken Salad

FAT RELEASERS: chicken, cucumber, tomato, oil, vinegar, strawberries
- **Phase 2:** Serve yourself the Oriental Chicken Salad with no dressing. Have 1 spoon of Cucumber Tomato Salad and 3 spoons of strawberries.
- **Phase 3:** Reduce the amount of chicken by 1 ounce, or about 2 tablespoons, and add 1 slice wheat bread.

Beef & Broccoli Stir-Fry

FAT RELEASERS: beef, broccoli, cantaloupe, honeydew, watermelon
• **Phase 2:** Dish out 2 spoons of the Beef & Broccoli Stir-Fry and 3 spoons of assorted melon.
• **Phase 3:** Reduce the amount of beef by 1 ounce, or about 2 tablespoons, and add ½ cup rice.

Chicken Zucchini Stir-Fry

FAT RELEASERS: chicken, zucchini, lettuce, veggies, orange
• **Phase 2:** Take 3 spoons of the Chicken Zucchini Stir-Fry. Have 2 cups of the Spring Mix, 4 spoons of assorted raw veggies, and 2 spoons of orange slices.
• **Phase 3:** Reduce the amount of chicken by 1 ounce, or about 2 table-spoons, and add ½ cup rice.

Oven Roasted Rotisserie Style Turkey

FAT RELEASERS: turkey, beans, vegetables, lettuce, sesame seeds
• **Phase 2:** Serve yourself 4 ounces of the Oven Roasted Rotisserie Style Turkey. Have 2 ladles (1 cup) of the Chili Bean Soup, 2 cups of Spring Mix, 4 spoons of assorted raw veggies, and 1 spoon of hummus.
• **Phase 3:** Reduce the amount of tur-key by 1 ounce, or about 2 tablespoons, and add ½ cup of vegetable rice pilaf.

Baked Fish

FAT RELEASERS: fish, lettuce, veggies, cucumber, tomato, oil, vinegar, orange
• **Phase 2:** Have 2 pieces of the Baked Fish, 2 cups of romaine lettuce, 4 spoons of assorted raw veggies, 1 spoon of Cucumber Tomato Salad, and 2 spoons of orange slices.
• **Phase 3:** Reduce the amount of fish by 1 ounce, or about 2 tablespoons, and add ½ cup of dirty rice.

Carved Salmon Fillet

FAT RELEASERS: salmon, lettuce, cucumber, tomato, oil, vinegar, orange
• **Phase 2:** Take 4 ounces of the Carved Salmon Fillet, plus 2 cups of the Spring Mix, 1 spoon of the Cucumber Tomato Salad, and 2 spoons of orange slices.
• **Phase 3:** Reduce the amount of salm-on by 1 ounce, or about 2 tablespoons, and add ½ plain baked potato.

Wood-Seared Salmon

FAT RELEASERS: salmon, lettuce, vegetables, beets, vinegar, grapes
• **Phase 2:** Have 4 ounces of the Wood-Seared Salmon, plus 2 cups of romaine lettuce, 4 spoons of assorted raw veggies, 1 spoon of pickled beets, and 1 spoon of grapes.
• **Phase 3:** Reduce the amount of salmon by 1 ounce, or about 2 table-spoons, and add ½ cup dirty rice.

SBARRO

● More than 1,000 locations

● (800) 456-GUEST; www.sbarro.com

The menu at Sbarro, a standard in shopping malls, is a bit limited for Digest Diet diners. We chose a couple of pasta dishes, without the pasta, plus an entrée salad.

Chicken Tenders with Mixed Vegetables

FAT RELEASERS: chicken, squash, broccoli, carrot

● **Phase 2:** Order the Chicken Tenders with Mixed Vegetables with no spaghetti.

● **Phase 3:** Reduce the amount of chicken by 1 ounce, or about 2 tablespoons, and add ½ cup Vegetable Rice.

Chicken Portofino

FAT RELEASERS: chicken, squash, lettuce, cucumbers, tomato, bell pepper, cabbage, carrot

● **Phase 2:** Order the Chicken Portofino with no spaghetti. Have a Garden Fresh Salad with no dressing.

● **Phase 3:** Reduce the amount of chicken by 1 ounce, or about 2 tablespoons, and add ½ cup spaghetti.

Greek Salad

FAT RELEASERS: spinach, onion, cheese, olives, zucchini, squash, broccoli, carrot, watermelon, cantaloupe, honeydew, strawberries, kiwi, grapes

● **Phase 2:** Order a Greek Salad with no dressing. Have 1 order of sautéed mixed vegetables and 1 order of a fruit salad.

● **Phase 3:** No change

SCHLOTZSKY'S DELI

- More than 350 locations in 35 states and 4 foreign countries
- (512) 236-3600; www.schlotzskys.com

Schlotzsky's has a standard deli sandwich menu with mostly sandwich fixings, plus pizzas, a few soups, and main course salads. For the most flexibility, create your own chef's salad from the various offerings, all of which are listed, with nutrition information, on the online menu.

> ### ● WARNING! Fat Increaser Ahead
> Breads and other grain foods made with white flour can destabilize blood sugar and contribute to weight gain. The story is different for whole grains—people who include whole grains in their diet tend to have a lower BMI and are less likely to develop diabetes, heart disease, and other illnesses.

Vegetable Beef & Barley Soup

FAT RELEASERS: vegetables, beef, barley
- **Phase 1:** Order 1 bowl of the Vegetable Beef & Barley Soup.
- **Phases 2 and 3:** No change

Vegetable Soup

FAT RELEASERS: tomato, beans, vegetables
- **Phase 1:** Order 1 bowl of Vegetable Soup.
- **Phases 2 and 3:** No change

Timberline Chili

FAT RELEASERS: beef, beans, bell pepper, tomato, lettuce, olives, chile pepper, cucumber
- **Phase 2:** Order 1 cup of the Timberline Chili. Have a Garden Salad with no dressing or bread and 2 ounces of Angus roast beef.
- **Phase 3:** No change

Chef Salad

FAT RELEASERS: lettuce, olives, chile pepper, cucumber, tomato, turkey, beef, chicken, avocado
• **Phase 2:** Order a Turkey Chef Salad with no dressing or bread. Ask to add 1 ounce of Angus roast beef, 1 ounce of chicken breast, and 1 scoop of guacamole.
• **Phase 3:** No change

Turkey Chef Salad

FAT RELEASERS: lettuce, turkey, cheese, olives, chile pepper, onion, tomato
• **Phase 2:** Order the Turkey Chef Salad with no dressing, bacon, or bread.
• **Phase 3:** No change

Cranberry, Apple, Pecan & Chicken Salad

FAT RELEASERS: chicken, lettuce, onion, apple, pecans, cheese, tomato, beans, vegetables
• **Phase 2:** Have ½ order of the Cranberry, Apple, Pecan & Chicken Salad with no dressing, cranberries, croutons, or bread. Have 1 bowl of the Vegetarian Vegetable Soup.
• **Phase 3:** No change

SIZZLER

- About 170 restaurants
- (949) 273-4497; www.sizzler.com

The Sizzler chain offers steakhouse fare in more modest portions. Special requests are no problem; in fact, they're encouraged. So you can feel comfortable ordering your meal exactly as you want it. Visit the salad bar for a variety of vegetable and protein options. The Sizzler website provides nutrition information, in food label format, on all menu items.

> **Fun Fat Fact**
>
> Vinegar has been shown to suppress body fat buildup in mice and is thought to do the same in humans.

Petite 6 oz. Tri-Tip

FAT RELEASERS: beef, broccoli
- **Phase 2:** Order the Petite 6 oz. Tri-Tip with broccoli and an extra order of broccoli.
- **Phase 3:** Reduce the amount of beef by 1 ounce, or about 2 tablespoons, and add ½ baked potato.

Chicken Chili

FAT RELEASERS: chicken, beans, tomato, lettuce, spinach, vegetables, turkey, cucumber, grapes
- **Phase 2:** Order 1 bowl of Chicken Chili. Have a salad with 4 serving tongs (1 cup) of lettuce or spinach, 4 tongs (1 cup) of fresh salad bar veggies, 3 small serving tongs (½ cup) of turkey ham, 1 serving spoon (½ cup) of Cucumber Tomato Salad, and 2 serving spoons (1 cup) of grapes.
- **Phase 3:** No change

Hibachi Chicken

FAT RELEASERS: chicken, cabbage, beans, grapes

• **Phase 2:** Order 1 single Hibachi Chicken. Have 4 serving spoons (2 cups) of Asian Chopped Salad with 2 small serving spoons (¾ cup) of Three Bean Salad and 2 serving spoons (1 cup) of grapes.

• **Phase 3:** No change

Grilled Salmon

FAT RELEASERS: salmon, vegetables

• **Phase 2:** Order the Grilled Salmon with the vegetable medley and no rice. Have 1 bowl of Garden Vegetable Soup.

• **Phase 3:** No change

Grilled Shrimp Skewers

FAT RELEASERS: shrimp, beans, vegetables, lettuce, spinach, beets, vinegar, egg, grapes

• **Phase 2:** Order the Grilled Shrimp Skewers with no broccoli, margarine, or rice. Have 1 bowl of Navy Bean Soup, 2 serving tongs (½ cup) of salad bar salad with fresh salad bar veggies, 2 tongs (½ cup) of lettuce or spinach, 1 tong (¼ cup) of pickled beets, 1 tong (¼ cup) of eggs, and 2 serving spoons (1 cup) of grapes.

• **Phase 3:** No change

● WARNING! Fat Increaser Ahead

Cutting both calories and portion size to lose weight can leave you overly hungry. Researchers at Penn State University discovered that including water-rich foods such as raw veggies, salad, and soup in your meal fills you up while helping you eat fewer calories.

SMOOTHIE KING

- More than 600 locations
- (985) 635-6973; www.smoothieking.com

The lone national smoothie chain with Digest Diet offerings, Smoothie King has a few standard smoothies that closely match Phase 1 guidelines for protein, fruit/fiber, and healthy fats. Ask to "make it skinny" to leave out the turbinado sugar. Check out the online menu before you go to explore other ingredient combinations.

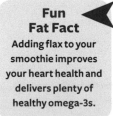

Fun Fat Fact

Adding flax to your smoothie improves your heart health and delivers plenty of healthy omega-3s.

Peanut Power

FAT RELEASERS: peanut, banana, milk, soy, honey
- **All phases:** Order a 20-ounce Peanut Power smoothie and ask to make it skinny.

Peanut Power Plus Strawberry

FAT RELEASERS: peanut, banana, strawberries, milk, soy, honey
- **All phases:** Order a 20-ounce Peanut Power Plus Strawberry smoothie and ask to make it skinny.

Coconut Surprise

FAT RELEASERS: coconut, pineapple, banana, milk, honey
- **All phases:** Order a 20-ounce Coconut Surprise smoothie and ask to make it skinny.

Piña Colada Island

FAT RELEASERS: pineapple, coconut, milk, honey
- **All phases:** Order a 20-ounce Piña Colada Island smoothie and ask to make it skinny.

STARBUCKS

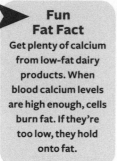

**Fun
Fat Fact**
Get plenty of calcium from low-fat dairy products. When blood calcium levels are high enough, cells burn fat. If they're too low, they hold onto fat.

● 17,000 retail stores in more than 55 countries
● (800) 782-7282; www.starbucks.com

The food items at Starbucks are prepackaged, so you don't have a lot of flexibility to change your meal. We picked a few meals that fit Phase 2 guidelines and paired several of them with coffee drinks that have milk and dairy. Starbucks changes its menu and updates its website frequently with menu and nutrition information.

Strawberry Smoothie

FAT RELEASERS: milk, strawberries, banana, protein powder, fiber powder
● **Phases 1 and 2:** Order a Grande (16 ounces) Strawberry Smoothie.

Chicken & Hummus Bistro Box

FAT RELEASERS: chicken, beans, cucumber, carrot, tomato, sesame seeds, cantaloupe, apple, grapes, blueberries, milk
● **Phase 2:** Order the Chicken & Hummus Bistro Box, but don't eat the pita. Have the Deluxe Fruit Blend Salad and an Iced Coffee made with nonfat milk.
● **Phase 3:** No change

Chipotle Chicken Wrap Bistro Box

FAT RELEASERS: chicken, cheese, cabbage, lime, tomato, avocado, cocoa, milk
• **Phase 2:** Order the Chipotle Chicken Wrap Bistro Box and skip the tortillas. Have a Grande (16 ounces) Cappuccino made with nonfat milk.
• **Phase 3:** No change

Protein Bistro Box

FAT RELEASERS: egg, cheese, honey, peanuts, apple, grapes, cantaloupe, blueberries
• **Phase 2:** Order the Protein Bistro Box. Have a Deluxe Fruit Blend Salad.
• **Phase 3:** No change

Cheese & Fruit Bistro Box

FAT RELEASERS: cheese, fruit, nuts, seeds
• **Phase 2:** Eat the Cheese & Fruit Bistro Box but skip the cranberries and crackers.
• **Phase 3:** Don't eat 1 piece of cheese and add 2 multigrain crackers from the Bistro Box in its place.

● WARNING! Fat Increaser Ahead

Order your coffee drink carefully. Any extras add either calories or fake ingredients that can increase fat. Always request fat-free (skim) milk, skip the whip, and say no to syrups of any kind. Instead, sprinkle your coffee with dashes of Digest Diet–friendly cocoa powder and cinnamon.

SUBWAY

- Close to 37,000 restaurants in 100 countries
- (203) 877-4281; www.subway.com

More than any other chain, Subway allows you to personalize your meal any way you like. You can mix and match lean proteins, add cheese if you wish, and choose any or all vegetables. You'll notice that we call for the amount of protein and veggies on the 12-inch sandwich to make sure that your meals include enough food. Subway's online nutrition info is comprehensive.

> **Fun Fat Fact**
> Scooping out a roll well removes about half the dough and half the calories.

Steak, Egg & Cheese Omelet

FAT RELEASERS: beef, egg, cheese, lettuce, tomato, onion, bell pepper, cucumber, olive, apple

- **Phase 2:** Order the Steak, Egg & Cheese Omelet with no bread, plus an extra order of steak, the Veggie Delite Salad with no dressing or croutons, and 1 package of apple slices.
- **Phase 3:** Reduce the amount of steak by 1 ounce, or about 2 tablespoons, and add ½ piece of a 6-inch 9-grain wheat bread.

Roast Beef Salad

FAT RELEASERS: beef, lettuce, tomato, onion, bell pepper, cucumber, olives, cheese, vegetables, apple

- **Phase 2:** Order the Roast Beef Salad and Veggie Delite Salad, no dressing or croutons on either, 1 extra order of roast beef, 1 slice of cheddar cheese, a 10-ounce bowl of Vegetable Beef Soup, and 1 package of apple slices.
- **Phase 3:** Eliminate the cheese, and add ½ of a 6-inch 9-grain wheat bread.

Black Forest Ham Salad

FAT RELEASERS: ham, lettuce, tomato, onion, bell pepper, cucumber, olives, avocado, vegetables, apple

• **Phase 2:** Order the Black Forest Ham Salad with no dressing or croutons. Have a Veggie Delite Salad with no dressing or croutons, topped with an extra order of avocado and 2 ounces of ham; also have a 10-ounce bowl of Minestrone Soup and a package of apple slices.

• **Phase 3:** Reduce the amount of ham by 1 ounce, or about 2 tablespoons, and add ½ of a 6-inch 9-grain wheat bread.

Turkey Breast & Black Forest Ham Salad

FAT RELEASERS: turkey, ham, lettuce, tomato, onion, bell pepper, cucumber, olives, vegetables, apple

• **Phase 2:** Make your own salad by combining the Turkey Breast & Black Forest Ham Salad with the Veggie Delite Salad, no dressing or croutons, plus an extra order of turkey breast. Then order a 10-ounce bowl of Minestrone Soup, and a package of apple slices.

• **Phase 3:** Reduce the amount of turkey by 1 ounce, or about 2 tablespoons, and add ½ of a 6-inch 9-grain wheat bread.

WARNING! Fat Increaser Ahead

Unlike their ultralean, protein-rich beef, ham, chicken and turkey fillings, Subway's Italian meats and meatballs are packed with calories coming mostly from fat.

Turkey Breast Salad

FAT RELEASERS: turkey, lettuce, tomato, onion, bell pepper, cucumber, olives, avocado, vegetables, beef

• **Phase 2:** Order the Turkey Breast Salad plus the Veggie Delite Salad with no dressing or croutons on either, plus 1 order of avocado, 1 order of turkey breast, and a 10-ounce bowl of Vegetable Beef Soup.

• **Phase 3:** Eliminate the avocado, and add ½ of a 6-inch 9-grain wheat bread.

Spinach Salad

FAT RELEASERS: spinach, egg, avocado, cheese, tomato, vegetables

• **Phase 2:** Make your own spinach salad with an egg patty, 1 order of avocado, 1 slice of Swiss cheese, and add a 10 ounces bowl of Minestrone Soup.

• **Phase 3:** Eliminate the cheese, and add ½ of a 6-inch 9-grain wheat bread.

Oven Roasted Chicken Salad

FAT RELEASERS: chicken, lettuce, tomato, onion, bell pepper, cucumber, olives, vegetables, beef, apple

• **Phase 2:** Order the Oven Roasted Chicken Breast Salad and combine it with a Veggie Delite Salad, without dressing or croutons, plus 1 order of chicken strips, a 10-ounce bowl of Vegetable Beef Soup and a package of apple slices.

• **Phase 3:** Reduce the amount of chicken by 1 ounce, or about 2 table-spoons, and add ½ of a 6-inch 9-grain wheat bread.

Grilled Chicken & Baby Spinach Salad

FAT RELEASERS: chicken, spinach, lettuce, tomato, onion, bell pepper, cucumber, olives, avocado, vegetables

• **Phase 2:** Order the Grilled Chicken & Baby Spinach Salad, topped with 1 chicken patty and 1 order of avocado, and have a 10-ounce bowl of Minestrone Soup.

• **Phase 3:** Reduce the amount of chicken by 1 ounce, or about 2 table-spoons, and add ½ of a 6-inch 9-grain wheat bread.

TACO BELL

- 5,600 restaurants
- (800) TACO BELL; www.tacobell.com

Digest Diet choices are extremely limited at this chain, which has been synonymous with Mexican fast food for decades. To maximize fat releasers during Phase 2, stick with salads made with chicken or beef, lettuce, tomato, and beans, topped with citrus salsa, and watch out for the classic Tex-Mex fat increasers that come standard with most orders—sour cream, lots of cheese, and chips. Cut back the protein and add a soft tortilla to turn the salad into a Phase 3 meal.

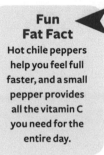

Fun Fat Fact

Hot chile peppers help you feel full faster, and a small pepper provides all the vitamin C you need for the entire day.

Fiesta Taco Salad

FAT RELEASERS: beef or chicken, lettuce, beans, tomato, citrus

- **Phase 2:** Order the Fiesta Taco Salad with citrus salsa and chicken, beef, or steak and without rice, tortilla strips, tortilla shell, and sour cream.
- **Phase 3:** Reduce the amount of chicken, beef, or steak by 1 ounce, or about 2 tablespoons, and add 1 soft tortilla.

● WARNING! Fat Increaser Ahead

Go for an early dinner rather than having a late-night fast-food meal. The food sitting in your stomach after eating late can prevent you from getting a good night's sleep, resulting in a shift in your hormone balance that causes your body to send hunger and eating signals.

T.G.I. FRIDAY'S

- More than 900 T.G.I. Friday's restaurants
- (800) FRIDAYS; www.tgifridays.com

**Fun
Fat Fact**

The vitamin C in foods such as tomatoes, broccoli, berries, and other vegetables and fruits helps speed up fat burning during exercise.

T.G.I. Friday's is a classic casual American-style restaurant with a variety of appetizers, entrées, burgers, and salads. The restaurant tries to accommodate special requests, so don't be shy about asking for modifications to the dishes you order. The T.G.I. Friday's menu provides nutrition information on all its menu offerings and updates frequently as the menu changes.

WARNING! Fat Increaser Ahead

You'd have to dance for hours to burn off the calories in a typical T.G.I. Friday's meal. If you bring along friends who like to share, it's easy to have fun while trimming calories.

Japanese Hibachi Black Angus Sirloin Tapa-tizer Skewers

FAT RELEASERS: beef, garlic, sesame seeds, broccoli, fruit

• **Phase 2:** Have ½ order of the Japanese Hibachi Black Angus Sirloin Tapa-tizer Skewers with 1 order of broccoli and 1 side order of fruit cup.

• **Phase 3:** Reduce the amount of steak by 1 ounce, or about 2 tablespoons, and add ½ cup Jasmine Rice Pilaf.

Mediterranean Black Angus Sirloin Tapa-tizer Skewers

FAT RELEASERS: beef, cucumber, yogurt, vegetables

• **Phase 2:** Have ½ order of the Mediterranean Black Angus Sirloin Tapa-tizer Skewers with no pita or slaw. Have 1 order of Fresh Vegetable Medley.

• **Phase 3:** Reduce the amount of steak by 1 ounce, or about 2 tablespoons, and add ½ cup mashed potatoes.

Strawberry Fields Salad with Grilled Balsamic Chicken

FAT RELEASERS: chicken, lettuce, strawberries, cheese, vinegar, broccoli, fruit

• **Phase 2:** Order the Strawberry Fields Salad with Grilled Balsamic Chicken with no dressing or pecans. Have 1 order of broccoli and 1 side order of fruit cup.

• **Phase 3:** Reduce the amount of chicken by 1 ounce, or about 2 tablespoons, and add 1 slice light rye bread.

Balsamic Glazed Chicken Caesar Salad

FAT RELEASERS: chicken, lettuce, cheese, tomato, vinegar

• **Phase 2:** Order the Balsamic-Glazed Chicken Caesar Salad with no dressing or croutons.

• **Phase 3:** Reduce the amount of chicken by 1 ounce, or about 2 tablespoons, and add 1 slice light rye bread.

UNO CHICAGO GRILL

● More than 150 restaurants
● (866) 600-8667; www.unos.com

I'm thrilled when I come across an Uno Chicago Grill in my travels. The menu has a lot of delicious choices that easily fit into Digest Diet guidelines. Protein portions tend to be large—you can try requesting a half portion, share half with a friend, or bring the leftovers home. Check out the online menu and nutrition information if you're in a position to plan ahead. Add brown rice or a piece of a whole-wheat bagel in Phase 3, or enjoy a slice of multigrain-crusted pizza.

Cuban Black Bean & Lentil Soup

FAT RELEASERS: beans, onion, chile pepper, orange, lettuce, avocado, broccoli
● **Phase 2:** Order 1 bowl of Cuban Black Bean & Lentil Soup with a side order of Citrus Avocado Salad with no dressing and 1 side order of steamed broccoli.
● **Phase 3:** No change

Top Sirloin Steak

FAT RELEASERS: beef, lettuce, tomato, cucumber, carrot, cabbage, avocado, onion
● **Phase 2:** Have ½ order of the Top Sirloin Steak. Have a side order of Roasted Seasonal Vegetables, 1 house salad with no dressing or croutons, and 2 tablespoons of guacamole with no chips.
● **Phase 3:** Reduce the amount of steak by 1 ounce, or about 2 tablespoons, and add ½ cup rice pilaf.

Chopped Honey Citrus Chicken Salad

FAT RELEASERS: chicken, lettuce, carrot, cucumber, peas, bell pepper, honey

• **Phase 2:** Order the Chopped Honey Citrus Chicken Salad with no dressing or tortilla strips.

• **Phase 3:** Reduce the amount of chicken by 1 ounce, or about 2 tablespoons, and add ½ scooped-out wholewheat bagel.

Chicken Caesar Salad

FAT RELEASERS: chicken, lettuce, cheese, vegetables

• **Phase 2:** Order the Chicken Caesar Salad with no dressing or croutons. Have 1 bowl of the Low-Fat Vegetarian Veggie Soup.

• **Phase 3:** Reduce the amount of chicken by 1 ounce, or about 2 tablespoons, and add ½ cup Red Bliss Mashed Potatoes.

Harvest Vegetable Five-Grain Thin Crust Pizza

FAT RELEASERS: bell pepper, whole grain, orange, lettuce, avocado, chicken

• **Phase 3 only:** Order 1 slice of the Harvest Vegetable Five-Grain Thin Crust Pizza. Have 1 side order of the Citrus Avocado Salad with no dressing and 4 ounces of grilled chicken breast.

Herb-Rubbed Breast of Chicken

FAT RELEASERS: chicken, orange, lettuce, avocado, broccoli, vegetables

• **Phase 2:** Have ½ order of the Herb-Rubbed Breast of Chicken. Have 1 side order each of steamed broccoli, steamed seasonal vegetables, and Citrus Avocado Salad with no dressing,

• **Phase 3:** Reduce the amount of chicken by 1 ounce, or 2 tablespoons, and add ½ cup brown rice.

Blackened Salmon

FAT RELEASERS: salmon, bell pepper, onion, tomato, lettuce, cheese, vegetables

• **Phase 2:** Have ½ order of the Blackened Salmon. Have 1 side order of a Caesar salad with no dressing or croutons and 1 side order of Roasted Seasonal Vegetables.

• **Phase 3:** Reduce the amount of salmon by 1 ounce, or about 2 tablespoons, and add ½ cup of brown rice.

WENDY'S

● More than 6,600 locations
● (614) 764-3100; www.wendys.com

One of the three traditional fast-food burger chains (McDonald's and Burger King are the others), Wendy's changes its menu—particularly its salads—often. Still, your best and most reliable options are a burger patty or grilled chicken paired with a side salad so that you don't have to deal with unwanted fat increasers in the main course salad. You won't find any whole grains on the Wendy's menu. The nutrition tool on the Wendy's website lets you adjust your meal and track the nutrition changes.

> **Fun Fat Fact**
> Low-fat and fat-free milk have the same amount of fat releasing calcium and protein as whole milk, for half to two-thirds of the calories.

● **WARNING! Fat Increaser Ahead**
The more often you eat fast food, the more likely you are to gain weight. Plus your risk of developing diabetes goes up. Here's the good news: Fast-food restaurants have increased their offerings of Digest Diet fare such as salads, grilled chicken, and fruit.

¼ Pound Hamburger Patty

FAT RELEASERS: beef, lettuce, tomato, onion, cheese, milk
● **Phase 2:** Order the ¼ Pound Hamburger Patty. Have an order of lettuce, tomato, and onion; 1 Caesar Side Salad with no dressing or croutons; and 1 TruMoo Lowfat White Milk.
● **Phase 3:** Add ½ bun.

Ultimate Chicken Grill

FAT RELEASERS: chicken, lettuce, tomato, onion, cheese, milk
● **Phase 2:** Order the Ultimate Chicken Grill with no bun or sauce. Have a Caesar Side Salad with no dressing or croutons and 1 TruMoo Lowfat White Milk.
● **Phase 3:** Reduce the amount of chicken by 1 ounce, or about 2 tablespoons, and add ½ bun.

Apple Pecan Chicken Salad

FAT RELEASERS: chicken, lettuce, apple, pecans, cheese, cranberries, milk
● **Phase 2:** Order the Apple Pecan Chicken Salad with no dressing or pecans. Have 1 TruMoo Lowfat White Milk.
● **Phase 3:** Reduce the amount of chicken by 1 ounce, or about 2 tablespoons, and add ½ bun.

Berry Almond Chicken Salad

FAT RELEASERS: chicken, lettuce, blueberries, strawberries, cheese, almonds, milk
● **Phase 2:** Order the Berry Almond Chicken Salad with no dressing and 1 TruMoo Lowfat White Milk.
● **Phase 3:** Reduce the amount of chicken by 1 ounce, or about 2 tablespoons, and add ½ bun.

The Digest Diet

*Keep track of Digest Diet meals
you find at your favorite restaurants here*

RESTAURANT	MEAL

RESTAURANT	MEAL

TheDigest Diet ®

Get everything you need to stay
slim for life!

Visit our online store and find unique ingredients, the best kitchen accessories, every book in the Digest Diet series, and so much more!

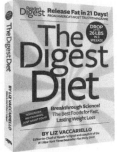

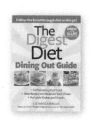

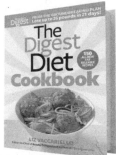

The Digest Diet
Jump-start weight loss and get your body into "fat release" mode.

The Digest Diet Dining Out Guide
Eat well anytime, anywhere with this handy pocket guide.

The Digest Diet Cookbook
Enjoy 150 NEW recipes to maintain weight loss and still enjoy every bite.

One-Click Shopping
All the essentials, shipped right to you! Shop for ingredients by each phase of the diet, plus handy travel containers, kitchen tools, accessories, and more.